Ocular
Therapeutics

Third Edition

Contributors

Kamna Verma MBBS, MS (Ophthalmology)
Research Associate
Dr RP Centre for Ophthalmic Sciences
All India Institute of Medical Sciences, New Delhi

Alok K Ravi MSc, PhD
Research Scholar
Ocular Pharmacology Division
Dr RP Centre for Ophthalmic Sciences
All India Institute of Medical Sciences, New Delhi

Shuchita Jhingan B Pharm
Pharmacist
Ocular Pharmacology Division
Dr RP Centre for Ophthalmic Sciences
All India Institute of Medical Sciences, New Delhi

Ocular Therapeutics

Third Edition

NR Biswas
MD (Pharmacology), DM (Clinical Pharmacology),
DNB (Clinical Pharmacology and Therapeutics), DSc

Professor, Department of Pharmacology
All India Institute of Medical Sciences, New Delhi

Viney Gupta
MD (Ophthalmology)

Associate Professor
Dr RP Centre for Ophthalmic Sciences
All India Institute of Medical Sciences, New Delhi

Ashok Dubey
DOMS, MD (Pharmacology)

Assistant Professor
School of Medical Sciences and Research
Sharda University, Greater Noida, UP

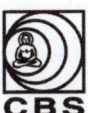

CBS

CBS Publishers & Distributors Pvt Ltd

New Delhi • Bengaluru • Chennai • Kochi • Kolkata • Mumbai
Bhopal • Bhubaneswar • Hyderabad • Jharkhand • Nagpur • Patna • Pune • Uttarakhand • Dhaka (Bangladesh)

Ocular Therapeutics

ISBN: 978-81-239-1959-1

Copyright © Authors and Publisher

Third Edition : 2011
 Reprint: 2019
Second Edition : 2004
First Edition : 2002

Published by Satish Kumar Jain and produced by Varun Jain for
CBS Publishers & Distributors Pvt Ltd
4819/XI Prahlad Street, 24 Ansari Road, Daryaganj, New Delhi 110 002, India.
Ph: 23289259, 23266861, 23266867   Fax: 011-23243014   Website: www.cbspd.com
                                    e-mail: delhi@cbspd.com; cbspubs@airtelmail.in.
Corporate Office: 204 FIE, Industrial Area, Patparganj, Delhi 110 092
Ph: 4934 4934   Fax: 4934 4935   e-mail: publishing@cbspd.com;
                                        publicity@cbspd.com

Branches

- **Bengaluru:** Seema House 2975, 17th Cross, K.R. Road,
  Banasankari 2nd Stage, Bengaluru 560 070, Karnataka
  Ph: +91-80-26771678/79   Fax: +91-80-26771680   e-mail: bangalore@cbspd.com
- **Chennai:** 7, Subbaraya Street, Shenoy Nagar, Chennai 600 030, Tamil Nadu
  Ph: +91-44-26680620, 26681266   Fax: +91-44-42032115   e-mail: chennai@cbspd.com
- **Kochi:** 42/1325, 1326, Power House Road, Opp. KSEB Power House
  Ernakulam 682 018, Kochi, Kerala
  Ph: +91-484-4059061-65   Fax: +91-484-4059065   e-mail: kochi@cbspd.com
- **Kolkata:** 6/B, Ground Floor, Rameswar Shaw Road, Kolkata-700 014, West Bengal
  Ph: +91-33-22891126, 22891127, 22891128   e-mail: kolkata@cbspd.com
- **Mumbai:** 83-C, Dr E Moses Road, Worli, Mumbai-400018, Maharashtra
  Ph: +91-22-24902340/41   Fax: +91-22-24902342   e-mail: mumbai@cbspd.com

Representatives

• Bhopal	0-8319310552	• Bhubaneswar	0-9911037372	• **Hyderabad**	0-9885175004
• Jharkhand	0-9811541605	• Nagpur	0-9021734563	• **Patna**	0-9334159340
• Pune	0-9623451994	• Uttarakhand	0-9716462459	• **Dhaka** (Bangladesh)	01912-003485

Printed at: India Binding House, Noida, UP

Foreword

In the last decade there has been a sea-change in the understanding of ocular pharmacodynamics. More and more drugs are being investigated as clinical trials in the management of ocular diseases like age-related macular degeneration, diabetic retinopathy, glaucoma, and so on. The emphasis is on non-invasive management of ophthalmic diseases and it would not be out of place if we understand that medical therapy would soon take centre stage of management of ophthalmic disorders.

Dr NR Biswas's first edition of *Ocular Therapeutics* was published in 2002. This is the third edition of the book in your hands. With the advent of anti-VEGF and other new drugs in the armamentarium of ophthalmologists, there has been a drastic change in the treatment algorithms. This book gives an insight into the recent developments in the field.

I hope this book written by Dr NR Biswas, Dr Viney Gupta and Dr Ashok Dubey will succeed admirably in meeting the aspirations of the readers who are looking for a book which can be used as a reference in their busy practice.

Prof Raj Vardhan Azad
Professor of Ophthalmology
Dr Rajendra Prasad Centre for
Ophthalmic Sciences
All India Institute of Medical Sciences
New Delhi, India

Message

My felicitations to Prof NR Biswas and his team for bringing out the third edition of *Ocular Therapeutics*.

This unique book concisely displays the contemporary and newer ophthalmic drugs and their actions, indications, contraindications and route of administration.

Written for the widest possible audience, I do believe that this book besides being of immense help to the students, teachers and practising ophthalmologists will also benefit personnel involved in National Programme for Prevention and Control of Blindness. Since pharmacology education is a borderless entity, this book should serve across India, Nepal and beyond.

I wish every success.

Prof PC Karmacharya MD
Vice Chancellor
BP Koirala Institute of Health Sciences
Dharan, Nepal

Preface to the Third Edition

The aim of this edition as that of the previous ones is to present drugs used in ophthalmology in an organized fashion. The book is intended as a ready-reckoner for an ophthalmologist as well as a student of ophthalmology. Compared to the past editions, the endeavour has been to focus on the clinically relevant aspects of ocular pharmacology, which a practising ophthalmologist faces in day-to-day practice.

Unfortunately, there are very few books on ocular pharmacology in India. We have tried to thoroughly update the book by the addition of the latest drugs in ocular pharmacology. We believe this book would be easy to read for the general ophthalmologist in a busy practice.

As advancement in pharmacology occurs with tremendous pace, there are a number of drugs which are no longer used and a huge number of new drugs have been recently introduced. We have tried to keep the book updated with the latest among ophthalmic drugs. Many new drugs especially among the topical nonsteroidal anti-inflammatory agents (NSAIDs) and antiallergic agents have been added. A new chapter on anti-VEGF agents has been incorporated while that on artificial tears has been removed, and it is now discussed with "other drugs".

There are subjects like drug delivery and gene therapeutics which have shown considerable advancement over the years. However, we have not included these in the book as the emphasis has been on clinical pharmacology.

We sincerely thank Dr Reena Sharma for helping write Chapter 9. Suggestions from the readers are welcome (gupta_v20032000@yahoo.com).

NR Biswas
Viney Gupta
Ashok Dubey

Preface to the First Edition

This book is the continuation of Formulary and Manual for the Production of Ophthalmic Drugs edited by Prof SK Gupta and Ms Shuchita Jhingan, which provided mainly information on the essential drugs and diagnostic adis. This formulary will provide reasonably comprehensive information on ophthalmic medications. It contains 18 chapters of different groups of ophthalmic drugs like antibiotics, topical steroids, NSAIDs, mydriatics, cycloplegics, antiglaucoma agents, immunosuppressives, etc. with indications, contraindications, warning, dosage, side effects, etc.

This manual, we are sure, may provide ready references and meet the growing needs of the family physicians, medical and BSc (Hons) ophthalmic techniques students, resident doctors and also practising ophthalmologists, particularly those who are posted in district hospitals and in primary health centres.

Suggestions for improvement from the readers are welcome.

NR Biswas

Contents

Ophthalmic Drugs and Materials

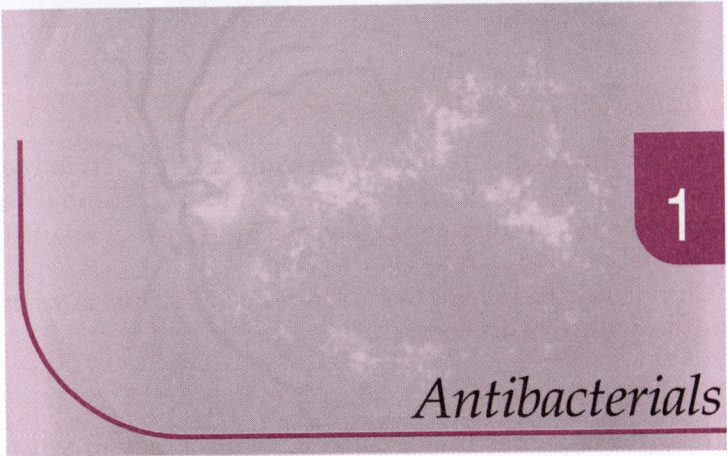

Antibacterials

CHLORAMPHENICOL AND POLYPEPTIDES

CHLORAMPHENICOL
(Mycin, Vanmycetin, Andrecin, Chlormet)

Description

Chloramphenicol is a broad-spectrum antibiotic originally isolated from *Streptomyces venezuelae*. It inhibits protein synthesis by interfering with the transfer of activated amino acids from soluble RNA to ribosome. It is bacteriostatic and binds reversibly to the 50S subunit of the bacterial ribosome. It is available as 1% sterile ointment.

Clinical Pharmacology

It is a highly lipophilic drug and penetrates the cornea well. The peak concentration of chloramphenicol is achieved in the aqueous humor within an hour of the drug application as drop or ointment. But generally these concentrations are below the minimum inhibitory concentrations required for many bacteria. So it should not be preferred in serious infections.

Indications

Chloramphenicol is indicated for the treatment of ocular infections involving the conjunctiva and cornea caused by chloramphenicol susceptible organisms. It is effective against both aerobic and anaerobic gram +ve and –ve organisms including rickettsiae. It is not active against *Chlamydia*.

It can be used in mild to moderate bacterial infections of lids, conjunctiva and cornea.

Adverse Reactions

Topical ophthalmic use of chloramphenicol may produce redness, itching, burning and stinging sensation. Less commonly, allergic reactions have also been reported of varying severity.

Contraindications

This product is contraindicated in persons sensitive to any of the components.

Precaution

Bone marrow hypoplasia including aplastic anemia and death has been reported following systemic administration. Chloramphenicol should not be used when less potentially dangerous agents would be expected to provide effective treatment. As a systemic drug it should be used only in those infections for which less potent drugs are ineffective or contraindicated.

The prolonged use of antibiotics may occasionally result in overgrowth of non-susceptible organisms including fungi. If new infections appear during medication, the drug should be discontinued and appropriate measures should be taken.

Dosage and Administration

- A small amount of ointment placed in the lower conjunctival sac every three hours or more frequently if deemed advisable by the prescribing physician. Treatment should be continued for at least 48 hours after the eye appears normal.

- Chloramphenicol eye drops should be instilled, one to two drops, 4 to 6 times daily. Treatment should generally be for one week.

POLYMYXIN B SULFATE
(Ocupol, Pychlor, Neosporin Eye, Oriprim-P)

Description

Polymixin B sulfate is a heptapeptide antibiotic derived from *B. aerosporus*. Sterile polymixin B is in powder form suitable for preparation of sterile solutions for intramuscular, intravenous drip, intrathecal or ophthalmic use. Each milligram of pure polymyxin B base is equivalent to 10,000 units of polymixin B and each microgram of pure polymixin B and base are equivalent to 10 units of polymyxin B.

For ocular infections polymyxin B preparations are available generally in combination with other antibiotics as Neomycin.

Actions

Polymyxin B sulfate has a bactericidal action against almost all gram-negative bacilli except the *Proteus* and *Nisseria* group. Polymyxins increase the permeability of bacterial cell membranes. They also have inhibitory actions on bacterial endotoxins.

Indications

When used systemically it has significant toxicity so its use is mainly in topical formulations. It is mainly used for bacterial infections of cornea and conjunctiva by susceptible organisms. Acute infections caused by resistant strains of *Pseudomonas aeruginosa* to other drugs have been seen to respond to Polymyxin.

Contraindications

This drug is contraindicated in persons with a prior history of hypersensitivity reactions to the polymyxin.

Warning

The safety of this drug in women during pregnancy has not been established.

Adverse Reactions

Local irritation, itching redness, and swelling may occur. The formulations generally contain polymyxin in combination with other drugs so long term use can also predispose to secondary viral and fungal infections.

Dosage and Administration

- *Ophthalmic:* Dissolve 500,000 units polymyxin-B sulfate in 20–50 ml sterile distilled water or sterile physiologic saline for 10,000–25,000 units per ml concentration. For the treatment of *Ps. aeruginosa* infections of the eye, a concentration of 0.1% to 0.25% (10,000–25,000 units per ml) is administered 1–3 drops every hour, increasing the intervals as response indicates.
- Combination products of polymyxin with neomycin, bacitracin and/or steroids are given one to two drops every 3 to 4 hours.

BACITRACIN

Description

Bacitracin is a bactericidal peptide antibiotic with a range of activity closely resembling that of penicillin. It is derived from *Bacillus subtilis*. In contrast to polymyxin it is active chiefly against gram-positive organisms but also affects Spirochetes, Gonococci, *Entamoeba histolytica* and *Actinomyces*. Bacitracin is ineffective against most gram-negative bacilli. Most gram-positive organisms are inhibited by 0.001 to 0.5 unit/ml of the drug. Although the antibacterial spectrum of bacitracin is comparable to that of penicillin, for topical ocular use, bacitracin is preferable to penicillin because fewer strains of organisms are resistant, allergy is less frequent and sensitization that prevents future use of penicillin is avoided. Bacitracin does not penetrate the cornea in therapeutic amounts.

Mechanism of Action

It acts by interfering with bacterial cell wall synthesis. It is available as zinc salt because zinc helps in the formation of bacitracin complex with bacterial structure.

Adverse Effects

Concentrations of 500 to 1000 units/g are non-irritating to the eye and other tissues and cause no undesirable systemic effects.

Precaution

Bacitracin solutions are unstable, but reasonable potency may be maintained for three weeks if the solution is refrigerated. The dry powder and ointment preparations are stable for over a year at room temperature. It is not to be used systemically.

AMINOGYCOSIDES

All aminoglycosides acts by binding to 30S subunit of bacterial ribosomal RNA and inhibiting protein synthesis. They are useful mainly against aerobic gram-negative bacteria and are bactericidal in nature.

GENTAMICIN

(Andregen, Genticin, Genoptic Liquifilm, Tamigen)

Description

Gentamicin sulfate is a water-soluble antibiotic of the aminoglycoside group active against a wide variety of pathogenic gram-negative and gram-positive bacteria. It is derived from *Micromonospora purpurea*.

Gentamicin sulfate is available as 0.3% drops or 3 mg/g ointment. *Spectrum*: The gram-positive bacteria against which gentamicin is active includes coagulase positive and coagulase negative staphylococci including certain strains that are resistant to penicillin. The gram-negative bacteria against which gentamicin is effective includes strains of *Pseudomonas aeruginosa, Proteus species, E. coli, Klebsiella pneumoniae, Haemophilus influenzae, Neisseria gonorrhoea,* etc.

Indications

Gentamicin is indicated in the topical treatment of infections of the external eye and its adnexa caused by susceptible bacteria. It is also used in irrigating fluids during intraocular surgery.

Contraindications

Gentamicin ophthalmic solution and ointment are contraindicated in patients with known hypersensitivity to any of its components.

Warning

Gentamicin eyedrops are not for injection. It should not be injected sub-conjunctivally nor should be directly introduced into the anterior chamber of the eye. Prolonged use may result in secondary infections.

Adverse Reactions

Transient irritation, punctate keratitis and delayed re epithelialization has been reported with the use of gentamicin used topically. Intravitreal gentamicin is known to cause macular infarction.

Dosage and Administration

- *Topical:* 0.3% concentration one to two drops four times daily. Fortified drops (20 mg/ml) can be formulated from intravenous preparations. Ophthalmic ointment is available as 0.3% conc.
- *Intravitreal:* 200–400 µg/0.1 ml
- *Sub-conjunctival:* 20 mg/ml
- *Parenteral:* 3.5 mg/kg/8 hourly (I/M or I/V)
- *Irrigating fluid:* 4 mg/500 ml.

AMIKACIN
(Aminogen)

Description

Amikacin is a semi synthetic aminoglycoside derived from kanamycin. Because of a chemical modification amikacin is protected from aminoglycoside inactivating enzymes and thus is preferred drug for treatment of gram-negative infections in which resistance to both gentamicin and tobramycin occurs.

Indications

As it is active against most gram-negative bacilli that are resistant to other aminoglycosides and is less toxic when injected intravitreally it has become the primary antibiotic for treatment of endophthalmitis along with vancomycin or cephalosporins.

Adverse Reactions

Same as that of gentamicin though nephrotoxicity is much less than gentamicin and tobramycin when used systemically.

Dosage and Administration

- *Topical:* It is available as 0.3% and 1% solution for topical use. Fortified drops (20 mg/ml) can be formulated from intravenous preparation.
- *Intravitreal conc.:* 0.4 mg/0.1 ml
- *Subconj:* 20 mg/ml
- *Parenteral:* 15 mg/kg/day (8–12 hourly).

TOBRAMYCIN
(Tobacin, Obra, Ibrex, Tozen)

Description

Tobramycin 0.3% is a sterile topical ophthalmic antibiotic formulation prepared specifically for topical therapy of external infections.

In vitro studies have demonstrated tobramycin to be active against susceptible strains of the following microorganisms: Staphylococci including *S. aureus and S. epidermidis* (coagulase-positive and coagulase-negative including penicillin-resistant strains), *Pseudomonas aeruginosa, Escherichia coli, Klebsiella pneumoniae, Proteus mirabilis, Haemophilus influenzae* and *H. aegyptius*. Bacterial susceptibility studies demonstrate that in some cases microorganisms resistant to gentamicin retain susceptibility to tobramycin. A significant bacterial population resistant to tobramycin has not yet emerged, however, bacterial resistance may develop upon prolonged use.

Adverse Reactions

Most frequently adverse reactions are hypersensitivity and localized ocular toxicity including lid itching, swelling and conjunctival erythema.

Dosage and Administration

- *Topical drops:* Available as 0.3% solution. Fortified drops(20 mg/ml) have a shelf life of 30 days. Instill one or two drops into the affected eye (s) every four hours.
- *Intravitreal:* 0.15–0.2 mg/0.1 ml
- *Subconjunctival:* 15 mg/ml
- *Parenteral:* 3.5 mg/kg/day 8 hourly.

Precaution

Tobramycin drops should not be used when wearing soft contact lenses. Do not use the drops after 1 month of opening the vial.

FRAMYCETIN
(Soframycin)

Description

Soframycin (framycetin sulfate) is available as 0.5% ointment and eyedrops.

Indications and Uses

Conjunctivitis, blepharitis, styes of bacterial origin, keratitits, corneal ulcers, prophylaxis following removal of foreign body, pre and post operatively in ocular surgery.

Contraindications

Soframycin is contraindicated in persons showing hypersensitivity to any of its components.

Dosage and Administration

2–3 applications, if used alone. One application of ointment at bed time if eyedrops have been used during daytime.

NEOMYCIN SULFATE—GRAMICIDIN
(Neosporin)

Description

Neomycin sulfate and gramicidin ophthalmic solution is a sterile aqueous preparation for use in the treatment of superficial external ocular infections.

It is effective against strains of *Proteus, Klebsiella, Staphylococcus aureus, E. coli, Haemophilus influenzae, Pneumococci, Diphtheria bacilli,* etc.

Indications and Usage

This product is indicated in the short-term treatment of superficial external ocular infections. Generally used in combination with polymixin B (5000 U/gm) and bacitracin (500 units/gm). Neomycin has also been used for treatment of acanthamoeba keratitis.

Warning

Neomycin sulfate causes cutaneous sensitization like itching, reddening and edema of the conjunctiva and eye lid. During long-term use of neomycin containing products, periodic examination for such signs is advisable.

Adverse Reactions

The most frequent adverse reactions are localized hypersensitivity including itching, swelling and conjunctival erythema. Local irritation on instillation has been reported. Prolonged application of neomycin containing ointment has resulted sometimes in severe allergic reactions.

Dosage and Administration

- *Drops:* 1–2 drops (0.17%) two to four times daily.
- *Ointment:* Apply the ointment (5 mg/gm) every 3–4 hours for 7–10 days depending on the severity of the infection.

TETRACYCLINES

TETRACYCLINE HYDROCHLORIDE
(Ointment-Tetracycline, Terramycin)

Description

Tetracycline HCl ophthalmic ointment contains 10 mg of tetracycline HCl per gram in an anhydrous lanolin petroleum base. It is a broad spectrum bacteriostatic antibiotic effective against many gram positive and negative bacteria including anaerobes and atypical microrganisms.

Indications

For treatment of superficial ocular infections susceptible to tetracycline HCl. For example, *Staphylococcus aureus, Streptococcus sp., N. gonorrhoea, D. pneumoniae, H. influenzae, Klebsiella pneumoniae, E. coli, B. anthracis.*

It is used in the treatment of trachoma (in conjunction with oral therapy).

Mechanism of Action

Tetracyclines act by inhibiting the bacterial protein synthesis by binding to 30S ribosomal RNA.

Contraindications

This product is contraindicated in persons who have shown hypersensitivity to any of its components.

Adverse Reactions

Dermatitis and allied symptomatology have been reported. If adverse reaction or idiosyncrasy occurs, discontinue medication and institute appropriate therapy.

Dosage and Administration

- *Topical:* Apply the ointment(1%) directly to the affected eye every 2 hours or more frequently as the severity of the infection and the degree of the response indicate.
- *Oral:* Severe or stubborn infections may also require oral therapy. For trachoma 250–500 mg every 6 hourly for 4 weeks.

SULFONAMIDES

SULFACETAMIDE SODIUM
(Albucid, Andremide, Phenosulf, Zincoren)

Description

Sulfacetamide sodium solution is available in three concentration—10%, 20% and 30% and as 6% ointment. Sulfacetamide sodium exerts a bacteriostatic effect against a wide range of gram-positive and gram-negative micro-organisms by restricting through competition with para-amino benzoic acid, the synthesis of folic acid, which bacteria require for growth. Sulpha drugs, however, do not show good efficacy if there is substantial muco purulent discharge.

Indications

Sulfacetamide is indicated for the treatment of conjunctivitis, corneal ulcers, blepharitis, etc. It attains high concentrations in the aqueous humor. It can also be used as an adjunct to systemic therapy for trachoma.

Contraindications

Contraindicated in individuals with known or suspected sensitivity to sulfonamides.

Adverse Reactions

Sulfacetamide sodium may cause local irritation, stinging and burning.

Dosage and Administration

Instill one drop into lower conjunctival sac every two hours or less frequently according to severity of infection.

CEPHALOSPORINS

CEFAZOLIN
(Azolin, Reflin)

Description

Like penicillin, cefazolin is bactericidal and inhibits the third stage of bacterial cell wall synthesis. Due to loss of peptidoglycan in the cell wall, the bacterial cell wall becomes defective and gets lysed. Cefazolin is a first generation cephalosporin.

Indications

Cefazolin is useful in the management of keratitis, endophthalmitis, and other eye infections caused by sensitive organisms. Topical cefazolin is an excellent adjunct to aminoglycosides in the treatment of infectious keratitis.

Adverse Effects

Cephalosporins are safe in suggested doses, however, it may cause g.i. disturbances such as nausea, vomiting, abdominal cramps. These drugs may cause nephrotoxicity when used in high doses.

Contraindications

Known hypersensitivity to cephalosporins/penicillins.

Dosage

- *Topical:* Fortified drops 50 mg/ml (shelf life 1 week)
- *Intravitreal:* 2.25 mg/0.1 ml (It is available as 500 mg powder)
- *Sub-conjunctival:* 50–100 mg/ml
- *Oral:* Dosage is 250 mg to 1 g every 6 hourly.

CEFTAZIDIME
(Ceftidin)

Description

It is a third generation cephalosporin. It has highly augmented activity against gram-negative bacteria including *Pseudomonas*. However, it is less active against gram-positive bacteria. It is not effective orally.

Indications

It is primarily used to treat endophthalmitis.

Adverse Effects

Similar to that of other cephalosporins

Dosage

- *Intravitreal:* 2.25 mg/0.1 ml. When administered with vancomycin both antibiotics should be given in separate syringes as precipitation may occur when they are given together.
- *Sub-conjunctival:* 100 mg/ml
- *Parenteral:* 1–2 gm/8–12 hourly

FLUOROQUINOLONES

The fluoroquinolones act by interfering with the bacterial DNA synthesis by inhibiting the bacterial enzymes topoisomerase-II (DNA gyrase) and topoisomerase-IV. They are bactericidal in nature. The initial fluoroquinolones introduced were more effective against mainly gram-negative organisms. The newer fluoroquinolones are also effective against gram-positive organisms.

NORFLOXACIN
(Norflox, Nordac, Normax, Norzen)

Description

Norfloxacin is a synthetic broad spectrum antibacterial agent supplied as a sterile isotonic solution for topical ophthalmic use.

There is no cross resistance between norfloxacin and other classes of antibacterial agents. Therefore, norfloxacin generally demonstrates activity against indicated organisms resistant to some other antimicrobial agents. Norfloxacin has in vitro activity against a broad spectrum of gram-positive and gram-negative aerobic bacteria. Compared to others fluoroquinolones norfloxacin is the least active of the fluoroquinolones against both gram-positive and negative organisms.

Indications

Commonly used in conjunctivitis, keratitis, infected corneal ulcer, blepharitis, dacryocystitis.

Adverse Reactions

Most common adverse reactions are local burning or discomfort, bitter taste. On systemic use nausea, headache and transient arthralgias may occur.

Dosage and Administration
• *Topical:* 1–2 drops (0.3%) 4 hourly.

- *Severe infections:* 2 drops every hour.
- *Oral:* 400 mg twice/day for 5 days

CIPROFLOXACIN
(Ciplox, Cifran, Quinobact, Zoxan)

Description

Ciprofloxacin HCl is a fluoroquinolone antibacterial active against a broad spectrum of gram-positive and gram-negative ocular pathogens. The bactericidal action of ciprofloxacin results from interference with the enzyme DNA gyrase which is needed for synthesis of bacterial DNA.

Indications and Usage

Bacterial infections of eye like blepharitis, corneal ulcer, stye, conjunctivitis.

Contraindications

A history of allergy to ciprofloxacin or any other component of the medication is a contraindication to its use.

Adverse Reactions

Most commonly reported adverse reaction was local burning or discomfort. In corneal ulcer studies with frequent administration of the drug white crystalline precipitates were seen in some patients. Skin rashes were reported in few cases.

Dosage and Administration

- *Topical drops:* Available in 0.3% concentration. One or two drops instilled into the conjunctival sac every two hours while awake for two days and one or two drops every four hours while awake for next five days.
- *Intravitreal conc.:* 150 µg in 0.1 ml
- *Subconjunctival:* 20–40 mg/ml

- *Parenteral:* 200–400 mg I/V twice/day (It is available as a 100 ml bottle containing 200 mg of ciprofloxacin).
- *Oral:* 500–700 mg/day 12 hourly.

OFLOXACIN
(Oflox, Oltaur, Zanocin, Exocin)

Description

Ofloxacin is a fluorinated carboxyquinolone antiinfective drug. Ofloxacin has in vitro activity against a broad range of gram-positive and gram-negative aerobic and anaerobic bacteria. Ofloxacin is bactericidal at concentrations equal to or slightly greater than inhibitory concentrations.

It acts by inhibiting DNA gyrase, an essential enzyme which is a critical catalyst in the duplication, transcription and repair of bacterial DNA.

Indications and Usage

Ofloxacin is used in the treatment of conjunctivitis caused by susceptible strains of the following bacteria: Gram-positive bacteria *Staphylococcus aureus, Staphylococcus epidermidis, Streptococcus pneumoniae.*

Gram-negative bacteria *Enterobacter cloacae, Haemophilus influenzae, Proteus mirabilis, Ps. aeruginosa.*

Contraindications

Ofloxacin is contraindicated in patients with a history of hypersensitivity to the drug or other quinolones.

Adverse Reactions

Incidences of ocular burning or discomfort are sometimes reported.

Other reactions may be stinging, redness, itching, photophobia, tearing and dry eyes.

Dosage and Administration

- *Local:* Instill one to two drops every two to four hours for the first two days and then four times daily in the affected eye.
- *Systemic:* 200–400 mg oral, twice/day.

LOMEFLOXACIN
(Okacin, Lomibact)

Description

It is a difluorinated quinolone derivative that is effective against both gram-positive and gram-negative bacteria. Cross resistance has been reported with other quinolones but not with any other group of antibiotics.

Precautions

Clinical studies of lomefloxacin drops during pregnancy and lactation are not available, hence should be used with caution in such cases. In order to avoid reduction of efficacy no ophthalmic preparation containing heavy metals such as zinc should be used 15 minutes preceding and following the use of lomefloxacin. It should be used within a month of opening the bottle.

Adverse Reactions

On systemic use rarely phototoxicity may occur.

Dosage and Administration

- *Ophthalmic solution:* 0.3 percent. A loading dose of one drop every 5 minutes for 20 minutes followed by twice a day for 7–9 days
- *Fortified drops:* 20 mg/ml (shelflife 15 days)
- *Subconjunctival dose:* 20–30 mg/ml
- *Oral dose:* 400 mg once daily for 5 days.

SPARFLOXACIN
(Scat, Zospar)

Description

It is a third generation fluroquinolone derivative with antibacterial activity against a wide range of gram-positive, gram-negative, atypical and anaerobic pathogenic bacteria.

Indications and Usage

External ocular infections such as conjunctivitis blepharitis dacryocystitis and acute meibomitis caused by susceptible bacteria.

Adverse Reactions

Ocular tolerance studies in rabbits have not revealed any severe intolerance reaction.

Contraindications

Hypersensitivity to quinolone group of antibacterials or any components of the preparation.

Precautions and Warning

If irritation or hypersensitivity to any component of the formulation develop, discontinue the use of the preparation and initiate appropriate therapy.

Dosage and Administration

Instill 1–2 drops in affected eye(s).

GATIFLOXACIN
(Gatiquin, Gate, Zymer, Gatiflox)

Description

It is a fourth generation fluoroquinolone.

Indications and Usage

Gatifloxacin has been found to be more effective than ciprofloxacin and levofloxacin for multiple drug resistant Staphylococci.

It is also effective against infection caused by anaerobic bacteria.

Adverse Reactions

Conjunctival irritation, increased lacrimation, papillary conjunctivitis.

Dosage and Administration

Topical: Available as 0.3% solution. One drop every two hourly initially for two days, then four hourly, depending on response, on the subsequent days.

LEVOFLOXACIN
(Levobact, Leeflox)

Description

Levofloxacin is a synthetic broad-spectrum antibacterial agent belonging to fluroquinolone group. It is available as 0.5% eyedrop. It is also available as oral tablet/solution and injection for systemic use.

Adverse Reactions

Blurred vision, stinging sensation, itching, swelling of the eyelid, bitter taste and photophobia can occur on topical levofloxacin application. Tendinopathy, tendon rupture, HSR reactions, hepatotoxicity, dizziness, convulsions, lightheadedness, diarrhea, peripheral neuropathy, prolongation of QT interval, phototoxicity and arthropathy are some of the concerns during sytemic levofloxacin therapy.

Precautions

As with any other broad-spectrum antibiotic there can be secondary infection with prolonged use of the drug. History of hypersensitivity to any quinolone is a contraindication for use. Systemic use is contraindicated in hepatic disease, epilepsy.

Indications and Usage

It can be used for treating the bacterial infections by susceptible *Staphylococcus*, *Streptococci*, *Corynebacterium*, *H.influenzae*, *Acinetobacter* and *Serratia*. Has also been found to be active against *Enterobacter*, *Legionella*, *Moraxella*, *Proteus*, *Providentia* and *Pseudomonas* in vitro.

Dosage and Administration

One to two drops are to be instilled every 2–6 hrs depending on the severity of the situation.

BESIFLOXACIN
(Besivance)

Description

Besifloxacin is a recently approved fourth generation fluoroquinolone antimicrobial drug for ophthalmic use only. It is available as 0.6% ophthalmic solution.

Pharmacology

Besifloxacin is an 8-chloro fluoroquinolone. Apart from inhibiting bacterial DNA gyrase and topoisomerase IV besifloxacin may also have antiinflammatory action as it has been shown to inhibit cytokine production by cytokines.

Indications and Usage

Besifloxacin ophthalmic solution is indicated for bacterial conjunctivitis caused by Staphylococci, Streptococci, *Moraxella*, *H.influenzae* and *Corynybacteria*. Because of the additional antiinflammatory effect it can of use in infections having inflammatory component.

Precautions

Prolonged use may result in super infection with growth of non-susceptible organisms. Contact lens use should be avoided during therapy.

Adverse Reactions

Conjunctival redness, pain, irritation/itching in the eye(s), blurred vision, and headache may occur.

Dosage and Administration

Besifloxacin should be administered three times daily for seven days.

MACROLIDES AND PEPTIDES

ERYTHROMYCIN
(Oral -Eltrocin, Erythrocin, E-Mycin, Erysafe)

Descriptions

It is bacteriostatic especially active against gram-positive bacilli, *Mycoplasma*, and *Chlamydia*. Because resistance develops fast among the gram-positive bacilli to macrolide antibiotics, they have limited use.

Mechanism of Action

Interferes with bacterial protein synthesis by binding to the 50S ribosomal subunit.

Indications

Erythromycin ointment can be used as a substitute to silver nitrate for the prophylaxis of ophthalmia neonatorum. It is as effective as tetracyclines for treating chlamydial infections and is safer in pregnant, nursing women and children < 8 years.

Precautions

Oral erythromycin estolate is not recommended for adults because of risk of cholestatic hepatitis.

Dosage

- *Topical:* It is dispensed as 0.3%–0.5% ointment
- *Oral dose:* 250–500 mg four times a day (depending on the salt form)

AZITHROMYCIN
(Oral-Azisara, Azithral, Aziwin, Aziwok)

Description

This macrolide is derived from erythromycin by adding methylated nitrogen. It has unique ability to act against intracellular pathogens like *Mycoplasma*, *Chlamydia* and *Legionella*. Compared to erythromycin it is more active against gram-negative bacteria such as *H influenzae* but less active against staphylococci and streptococci. As it has an extended half-life, its once daily dosing improves patient compliance. Mechanism of action is same as erythromycin.

Indications

It is a better effective treatment for trachoma when used orally because of difficulty of patient compliance with conventional treatment. Studies have also suggested that it may be used to effectively treat *Toxoplasma* infection.

Precautions

Concurrent administration of macrolides and astemizole or terfenadine can cause elevated antihistamine levels that can result in life-threatening arrhythmias.

Dosage

- 500 mg–1 gm once daily (taken preferably on empty stomach) for 3 days in chlamydial infections. Dose in children is 20 mg/kg body weight.

CLARITHROMYCIN
(Oral -Acem, Biclar, Celex, Clamycin)

Description

Clarithromycin is a methyl derivative of erythromycin with improved oral absorption. It is 10–50 times more potent than erythromycin and 40–50 times more potent than Azithromycin. Its mechanism of action is similar to erythromycin.

Adverse Effects

It has lower incidence of gastrointestinal side effects compared to erythromycin. Pseudomembranous colitis, and anaphylaxis have been reported.

Dosage

250 mg–500 mg twice a day for a week or 1000 mg of the extended release formulation once daily.

VANCOMYCIN
(Vancocin)

Description

It is a unique glycopeptide structurally unrelated to other antibiotics. It is bactericidal for most gram-positive organisms. Vancomycin acts by inhibiting cell wall synthesis. It is useful for staphylococcal infection non responsive to cephalosporins, methicilin resistant *Staphylococcus* and *Streptococcus viridans*.

Indications

Because of its excellent activity against gram-positive bacteria vancomycin is especially recommended for topical, sub-conjunctival and intravitreal therapy of bacterial endophthalmitis. It is also used in the irrigating fluid for intraocular surgery.

Adverse Effects

Vancomycin in large doses given systemically especially with other ototoxic and nephrotoxic drugs can cause permanent deafness and fatal uremia.

Precautions

If given parenterally, dosage must be adjusted in elderly patients who already have compromised glomerular filtration and thus need lower doses.

Dosage

- *Topical drops:* Fortified drops are dispensed as 50 mg/ml. However since the solution is acidic buffering is needed.
- *Intravitreal conc.:* Is 1 mg/0.1 ml
- *Sub-conjunctival:* 25 mg/ml
- *Parenteral:* 2 grams/6–12 hourly.
- After reconstitution with sterile water the vancomycin vials can be stored in a refrigerator for 14 days without loss of potency. However, if reconstituted with Ringer lactate or Dextrose saline its shelf life is reduced to 96 hours.
- *Irrigating fluid:* 10 mg/500 ml

METRONIDAZOLE
(Metrogyl, Aristogyl, Flagyl, Monizole)

Description

It is a 5 nitro imidazole derivative. It is a potent bactericidal agent effective against most anaerobic bacteria like *B fragilis, Clostidia, anaerobic Streptococci,* and *Peptococcus sp.*

Indication

Orbital cellulitis.

Adverse Reactions

Peripheral neuropathy, GI disturbance, metallic taste, headache, pruritis.

Dosage

- *Oral:* 400–800 mg every 8 hour
- *Intravenous:* 15 mg/kg infusion over 30–60 minutes.

Antiviral Agents

IDOXURIDINE
(Ridinox, Idurin, Toxil)

Description

Idoxuridine is a topical antiviral chemotherapeutic agent available as 0.1% drop and 0.5% ointment.

Actions

In chemical structure idoxuridine closely approximates the configuration of thymidine, one of the four building blocks of DNA–the genetic material of the herpes virus. As a result idoxuridine is able to replace thymidine in the enzymatic step of viral replication or 'growth'. The consequent production of faulty DNA results in a pseudo structure which cannot infect or destroy tissue.

Indications

For the treatment of keratitis caused by herpes virus.

Contraindications

Hypersensitivity to the active ingredient or other components of this medication.

Warning

Idoxuridine should be administered with caution in pregnancy because it has been reported to cross the placental barrier.

Idoxuridine has been reported to cause chromosome aberrations in mice and to be mutagenic in mammalian cells in culture. This cytotoxic drug should be regarded as being potentially carcinogenic. It can inhibit DNA synthesis or function and is incorporated into the DNA of mammalian cells as well as into the genome of DNA viruses.

Precautions

Some strains of herpes simplex virus appear to be resistant to the action of idoxuridine. If there is no lessening of fluorescein staining in 14 days, another form of medication should be undertaken. Recurrence may occur if medication is not continued 5 to 7 days after the lesion has healed.

Adverse Reactions

Occasional irritation, pain, pruritis, inflammation, edema of the eyes or lids, allergic reactions, photophobia, occasional corneal clouding, punctate defects in the corneal epithelium.

Dosage and Administration

For optimal results the infected tissues should be kept saturated with idoxuridine.

Instill one drop in the infected eye every hour during the day. At night the dosage may be reduced to one drop every other hour.

TRIFLUOROTHYMIDINE

Description

Trifluorothymidine 1% is a halogenated pyrimidine nucleoside. It is an antiviral drug for topical treatment of epithelial keratitis caused by herpes virus. Some strains of adenovirus are also inhibited in vitro.

Mechanism of Action

Trifluorothymidine interferes with DNA synthesis in cultured mammalian cells. Systemic absorption of trifluorothymidine following therapeutic doses appears to be negligible. No detectable concentrations of trifluoro-thymidine were found in the sera of adult healthy normal subjects who had trifluorothymidine instilled into their eyes seven times daily for 14 consecutive days.

Indications and Usage

Trifluorothymidine 1% is indicated for the treatment of primary viral keratoconjunctivitis and recurrent epithelial/stromal keratitis due to herpes simplex virus type 1 and type 2. Trifluorothymidine is also effective in the treatment of epithelial keratitis that has not responded clinically to the topical administration of idoxuridine or when ocular toxicity or hypersensitivity to idoxuridine has occurred.

Contraindications

Trifluorothymidine 1% ophthalmic solution is contraindicated for patients who develop hypersensitivity reactions or chemical intolerance to trifluorothymidine.

Precautions

Mutagenic potential: Trifluorothymidine has been shown to exert mutagenic effect. DNA damaging and cell transforming activities are seen in various standard in vitro test systems. The drug should not be prescribed for pregnant women unless the potential benefits outweigh the harmful effects.

Adverse Reactions

The most frequent adverse reactions reported during controlled clinical trials are mild, transient burning or stinging upon instillation and palpebral edema. Other adverse reactions reported were superficial punctate keratopathy, stromal edema, irritation, keratitis, hyperemia, and increased intraocular pressure.

Dosage and Administration

Instill one drop of trifluorothymidine ophthalmic solution 1% on to the cornea of the affected eye every two hours for a maximum daily dosage of nine drops daily until the corneal ulcer has completely re-epithelialized. Following re-epithelialization, instill one drop every four hours for additional seven days.

ACYCLOVIR
(Oint—Eye–Acivir, Acyclovir, Ocuvir)
(*Skin—Acivir, Cyclovir, Ocuvir, Herprex, Herperax*)
(Oral—Acivir, Cyclovir, Ocuvir, Herprex, Herperax)

Description

Acyclovir 3% is an acyclic nucleoside analogue with highly potent and specific activity against herpes simplex virus type 1 and 2 and herpes zoster. It is ten times more active against HSV-1 and HSV-2 than against VZV.

Pharmacology

Acyclovir is 10 to 20% available in plasma after oral administration. The bioavailability decreases with increasing dose. It has 9 to 33% plasma protein binding. The plasma half-life of acyclovir is 2.5 to 3 hours. It is excreted by glomerular filtration and tubular secretion. The half-life increases if there is renal dysfunction.

Food does not interfere the absorption of acyclovir so can be given unrelated to food. Cautious use is needed in patients with compromised renal function.

When given as eye ointment , therapeutic concentration is reached in aqueous humor quickly after absorption through corneal epithelium and other superficial structures. Systemic levels in blood after topical administration and in urine are insignificant.

Mechanism of Action

Viral and cellular thymidine kinase differ slightly from each other. Acyclovir can function as a substrate for viral thymidine kinase but not for cellular thymidine kinase. Thus, Acyclovir can enter the sequence of DNA formation only in cells infected by virus. The drug is transformed into acyclovir monophosphate, diphosphate and triphosphate. Acyclovir triphosphate inhibits viral DNA polymerases. It also gets incorporated into the viral DNA and causes chain termination.

Indications

Used for topical therapy of herpes simplex viral keratitis. It is superior to other antivirals in that it has deeper corneal penetration. Systemically it is used in herpes zoster ophthalmicus and acute retinal necrosis due to viral retinitis. For herpes zoster ophthalmicus, therapy should be started within 72 hours of the appearance of rash.

Contraindications

Contraindicated in persons having hypersensitivity to acyclovir.

Adverse Reactions

Local: Transient mild stinging immediately following administration occurs in few of patients. Superficial punctate keratopathy has been reported but this has not resulted in patients withdrawing from therapy and has healed without sequelae.

Systemic: On systemic use there may be nausea, vomiting, headache, anorexia, dizziness and fatigue. Intravenous use can potentiate nephrotoxicity. It should be administered in reduced doses in patients with renal impairment.

Dosage and Administration

- *Topical:* It is available as 3% ointment to be administered five times/day or as prescribed by the physician for 14–21 days.
- *Intravitreal dose:* 10–40 micrograms/0.1 ml
- Systemic: In acute HZO it is administered as 800 mg, 5 times daily for 7–10 days. For prophylaxis 400 mg 2 times daily for up to 12 months, followed by re-evaluation.

- *Parenteral:* In viral retinitis intravenous Acyclovir is administered (10 mg/kg infused at a constant rate over 1 hour, every 8 hours for 7–10 days) followed by an oral dose of 2–4 gm/day.
- Acyclovir sodium powder should be stored in tight light resistant container at 15–20°C. It should not be reconstituted with diluents containing parabens as precipitation may occur.

VIDARABINE
(Viva-A)

Description

Vidarabine ointment 3% is used as an antiviral drug for the topical treatment of keratitis caused by herpes simplex virus.

Clinical Pharmacology

Vidarabine is a purine nucleoside obtained from fermentation cultures of *Streptomyces antibioticus*. It possesses in vitro and in vivo activity against herpes simplex types 1 and 2, varicella zoster and vaccinia viruses.

Indications and Usage

Vidarabine ophthalmic ointment is indicated for the treatment of acute keratoconjunctivitis and recurrent epithelial keratitis due to herpes simplex virus type 1 and 2. It is also effective in superficial keratitis caused by herpes virus which has not responded to topical idoxuridine or when toxic or hypersensitivity reactions to idoxuridine have occurred.

Contraindications

Vidarabine is contraindicated in patients who develop hypersensitivity reactions to it.

Adverse Reaction

Lacrimation, foreign body sensation, conjunctival infection, burning, irritation, superficial punctate keratitis, pain, photophobia, punctal occlusion and sensitivity has been reported.

Dosage and Administration

Administer approximately half an inch of vidarabine ophthalmic ointment (3%) into the lower conjunctival sac five times daily at three hour intervals.

GANCICLOVIR
(Cytovene)

Description

It is an acyclic nucleoside analog of oxyguanosine. Ganciclovir is phosphorylated to ganciclovir triphosphate by cellular kinases in infected cells. The activated compound inhibits the viral DNA polymerase and causes termination of DNA chain elongation.

Indications and Usage

It has been used almost exclusively for Cytomegalovirus (CMV) retinitis. Compared to acyclovir, it is 10–25 times more effective against CMV. It has also been used to treat progressive outer retinal necrosis.

Adverse Effects

Myelosuppression develops in 25% patients. Nephrotoxicity and elevation of liver enzymes is reported. Adequate hydration of the patient is needed to avoid nephrotoxicity when administering ganciclovir.

Contraindications

Pregnant women and those who show hypersensitivity to ganciclovir.

Dosage

- *Oral:* 10 mg/kg body wt/dose 4–5 times/day

- *Intravenous:* 5 mg/kg over 1 hour every 12 hours for 14–21 days. It is available in lyophilized 500 mg vials to be reconstituted with sterile water.
- *Intravitreal:* 200–400 µg/0.1 ml. Before injection the solution should be filtered through a micropore filter. The injections are to be given twice weekly for 2–3 weeks or until the retinitis regresses.
- *Ganciclovir implant:* It consists of a 6 mg pellet of ganciclovir covered with polyvinyl alcohol releasing 1 µg/hour of ganciclovir. The implant has been shown to be more effective in delaying the progression of retinitis than systemic administration. It is replaced after 5 to 8 months.

VALACYCLOVIR
(Valavir, Valcivir)

Description
Valacyclovir is available as 500 mg or 1 g tablet for oral administration.

Pharmacology
Valacyclovir is a prodrug of acyclovir with more oral bioavailability. Antiviral activity is because of viral DNA polymerase inhibition thus arresting the growth of viral DNA. It is mainly effective against HSV types 1 (HSV-1) and 2 (HSV-2) and VZV.

Indications and Usage
For herpes zoster it is given 1 gram three times daily for seven days.

Adverse Effects
Headache, nausea, and abdominal pain are the most common adverse effects reported.

Precautions

Thrombotic thrombocytopenic purpura/hemolytic uremic syndrome, acute renal failure, and central nervous system adverse reactions (agitation, hallucinations, confusion, delirium, seizures, and encephalopathy) should be watched for, especially in elderly patients and those with impaired renal function. It is contraindicated in patients with history of hypersensitivity to valacyclovir, acyclovir, or any component of the formulation.

Dosage

The recommended dosage for treatment of herpes zoster is 1 gm 3 times daily for 7 days. Therapy is to be initiated early because it is most effective when started within 48 hours of the onset of rash.

FAMCICLOVIR
(Famtrex, Virovir)

Description

This antiviral is available as 125 mg, 250 mg or 500 mg tablets. It is not available for topical use.

Pharmacology

Famciclovir is a prodrug of penciclovir with better oral bioavailability. It inhibits viral DNA polymerase, consequently selectively inhibiting, viral DNA synthesis and replication.

Indications and Usage

It is effective against HSV-1, HSV-2 and varicella zoster infection. It may be used for the treatment of acute herpes zoster.

Precautions

Should be used with caution in patients with underlying renal disease.

Adverse Reactions

Headache, nausea and mild fever are the more common side effects. Acute renal failure is cautioned in at risk patients with underlying renal disease.

Dosage and Administration

Famciclovir is taken 500 mg three times a day for seven days. Treatment should be begun immediately after diagnosing herpes zoster as efficacy is not well established for drug taken 72 hours after the rash has appeared.

VALGANCICLOVIR
(Valcept, Valgan)

Description

This antiviral is available as 450 mg tablets. It is also available as powder for oral suspension which when constituted has 50 mg/ml of valganaciclovir drug base.

Pharmacology

Valganciclovir is a prodrug of ganciclovir that exists as a mixture of two diastereomers. After oral administration, both diastereomers are rapidly converted to ganciclovir by intestinal and hepatic enzymes. Being a prodrug of ganciclovir with higher bioavailability it has been seen that 900 mg of valgancyclovir provides a ganciclovir exposure (AUC) comparable to IV ganciclovir 5 mg/kg which is about 3000 to 3500 mg ganciclovir for adult. Ganciclovir is a synthetic analogue of 2'-deoxyguanosine, which inhibits replication of human cytomegalovirus in cell culture and in vivo by inhibiting viral DNA polymerase.

Indications and Usage

It is recommended for use in cytomegaloviral infections of eye such as CMV retinitis.

Adverse Reactions

Diarrhea, pyrexia, nausea, tremor, neutropenia, anemia, thrombocytopenia, and vomiting have been reported.

Contraindications

Hypersensitivity to valganciclovir or ganciclovir.

Dosage and Administration

Induction dose of 900 mg (two 450 mg tablets) twice a day for 21 days is followed by the maintenance dose of 900 mg (two 450 mg tablets) once a day.

FOSCARNET
(Foscavir)

Description

Foscarnet is an antiviral drug available as 24 mg/ml solution for intravenous injection.

Pharmacology

Foscarnet inhibits the viral replication by selectively inhibiting the pyrophosphate binding site on virus-specific DNA polymerases. It inhibits the cytomegalovirus (CMV) and herpes simplex virus types 1 and 2 (HSV-1 and HSV-2).

Indications and Usage

Foscarnet is indicated for the treatment of CMV retinitis in patients with acquired immunodeficiency syndrome (AIDS). Combination therapy with foscarnet and ganciclovir is given in patients who have relapse of CMV retinitis after monotherapy with either drug.

Precautions

Renal impairment is the major toxicity which can be precipitated in a predisposed patient. Serum electrolyte changes and seizures may also occur.

Adverse Reactions

Fever, nausea, vomiting, diarrhea and headache are the commonly associated adverse effects. The major toxicity of foscarnet is renal impairment.

Dosage and Administration

Foscarnet infusion 90 mg/kg (over 1–1/2 to 2 hour) every twelve hours or 60 mg/kg (over one hour) every eight hours, is given over 2–3 weeks depending on clinical response. Following induction, the maintenance dose of foscarnet for CMV retinitis is 90 mg/kg/day to 120 mg/kg/day (depending upon renal function) administered as infusion over 2 hours.

The standard solution may be used with or without dilution when using a central venous catheter for infusion. When infused through a peripheral vein, the solution is to be diluted to half the strength with 5% dextrose in water or with a normal saline solution prior to administration to avoid injection site reactions.

CIDOFOVIR
(Vistide)

Description

This injectible antiviral is available in a vial containing 375 mg of cidofovir in 5 ml aqueous solution at a concentration of 75 mg/ml.

Pharmacology

Cidofovir gets incorporated in the growing viral DNA chain and inhibits the viral DNA polymerase. This causes inhibition of viral DNA synthesis.

Indications and Usage

It is used for the treatment of CMV retinitis. It is also efficacious in delaying the progression of CMV retinitis in patients not responding to previous therapies.

Precautions

Renal function status should be confirmed before beginning the therapy because it is a nephrotoxic drug. Direct intraocular injection is contraindicated.

Adverse Reactions

Nephrotoxicity is the major concern. Proteinuria, nausea, vomiting, rash, neutropenia, fever, diarrhea, infection, alopecia, decreased intraocular pressure, anterior uveitis, and metabolic acidosis may occur.

Dosage and Administration

Induction dose is 5 mg/kg body weight intravenous infusion given over 1 hr administered once weekly for two consecutive weeks. Maintenance therapy is with the same dose but given once in two weeks.

FOMIVIRSEN
(Vitravene)

Description

Fomivirsen is available as an intravitreal injection in a concentration of 6.6 mg/ml to treat cytomegalovirus retinitis (CMV).

Pharmacology

Formiversen inhibits the CMV replication by binding to the viral mRNA and altering the regulation of viral gene expression.

Indications and Usage

It is used for treatment of CMV retinitis in immunocompromised patients where other drugs have not produced proper response or are contraindicated.

Adverse Reactions

Different inflammatory reactions in the eye, blurred vision, cataract, conjunctival hemorrhage, decreased visual acuity, eye pain, floaters, increased intraocular pressure, photophobia, retinal detachment and retinal pigment changes have been reported.

Precaution

Recent (2–4 weeks) history of cidofovir injection increases the chance of ocular inflammation.

Dosage and Administration

Initially 330 µg (0.05 ml) formivirsen injections are given once every two weeks for two doses. Then the maintenance dose is administered once every four weeks.

3

Antifungal and Antiparasitic Agents

NATAMYCIN
(Pimafucin)

Description

Natamycin is a 5% sterile, antifungal drug for topical ophthalmic administration.

Although the activity against fungi is dose related natamycin is predominantly fungicidal.

Clinical Pharmacology

Natamycin is a tetraene polyene antibiotic derived from *Streptomyces natalensis*. It possesses in vitro activity against a variety of yeast and filamentous fungi, including *Candida, Aspergillus, Cephalosporium, Fusarium* and *Penicillium*. The mechanism of action appears to be through binding of the molecule to the sterol moiety of the fungal cell membrane. The polyene sterol complex alters the permeability of the membrane to produce depletion of essential cellular constituents. Topical administration produces effective concentration of natamycin within the corneal stroma but not in the intraocular fluid. Natamycin is not absorbed from the gastrointestinal tract.

Indications and Usage

Natamycin is indicated for treatment of fungal blepharitis, conjunctivitis and keratitis caused by susceptible organisms. Natamycin is the initial drug of choice in *Fusarium keratitis*.

Contraindications

Natamycin is contraindicated in individuals with a history of hypersensitivity to any of its components.

Adverse Reactions

Conjunctival chemosis and hyperemia, thought to be allergic in nature may be seen in some individuals.

Dosage and Administration

The preferred initial dosage in fungal keratitis is one drop of natamycin instilled in the conjunctival sac at hourly or two hourly intervals. The frequency of application can be reduced to 6–8 times daily after the first 3–4 days. Therapy should generally be continued for 14–21 days. It is available as a suspension which can adhere to areas of epithelial ulceration.

NYSTATIN
(Nystatin)

Description

Nystatin is also a polyene antibiotic derived from *Streptomyces noursei* highly active in inhibiting the growth of a wide variety of fungi, moulds and yeasts. Nystatin is fungistatic, not fungicidal. Because of high systemic toxicity it is used only topically.

Mechanism of Action

The fungistatic action is due to the formation of polyenesterol complexes which render the fungal membrane leaky.

Indications

Used in therapy of *Aspergillus fumigatus* and *Candida albicans* keratitis. *Aspergillus* growth is inhibited by a nystatin concentration of 6–12 units/ml.

Adverse Effects

Nystatin produces few ocular side effects.

Uses and Dosage

Although not commercially available as an ocular medication, the dermatologic cream preparation can be used for keratitis. Topical application of nystatin ointment 100,000 units/g is of value in the treatment of external ocular infections caused by *Candida* or *Aspergillus*.

AMPHOTERICIN B
(L-AMB, AmBisome, Fungizone)

Description

Amphotericin B is an antifungal polyene antibiotic derived from a strain of *Streptomyces nodusus*. Amphotericin B is fungistatic rather than fungicidal in concentrations available in body fluids.

Mechanism of Action

It probably acts by binding to sterol in the fungus cell membrane with a resultant change in membrane permeability which allows leakage of intracellular components. Mammalian cell membrane also contain sterols and it has been suggested that the damage to human cells (toxicity) and damage to fungal cells (antibiotic effect) may share common mechanisms.

Indications

Amphotericin B is used in the treatment of corneal ulcers caused by a wide variety of fungi. Hourly instillation for the cure of mycotic keratitis caused by *Curvalaria lunata, Penicillium spimulosum, Gibberella fujkaroi, Fussidium terricola and Aspergillus sp.* is recommended. It is also used in treatment of intraocular histoplasmosis. In *Candida* keratitis, Amphotericin B is the most effective of all antifungals available topically. However, penetration through the intact cornea is better with natamycin than amphotericin.

Caution

Under no circumstances should a total daily dosage of 1.5 mg/kg be exceeded. The vial should be kept in a dark room as it is degraded in light. It is unclear whether frequent topical use results in elevated systemic levels and worsening of renal function tests in patients with nephrotoxicity.

Contraindications

Contraindicated in patients with nephropathy and in those persons showing hypersensitivity to amphotericin B.

Adverse Effects

When used systemically amphotericin B may produce local irritation (thrombophlebitis may occur in the injected vein), nausea, vomiting, diarrhoea and hematopoietic abnormalities (such as anemia, agranulocytosis and eosinophilia). In addition amphotericin B can cause renal damage which generally is reversible unless the total dose exceeds 3 gm. Nephrotoxicity is reported to occur in 80% patients on amphotericin. The liposomal preparations have fewer side effects.

Dosage and Administration

- *Topical:* A concentration of 0.15% is prepared from amphotericin B injection for topical use.
- Intravitreal/intracameral dose is 5–10 microgram/0.1 ml.
- *Subconjunctival:* Dose for subconjunctival injection is 0.5 mg to 1 mg.

- *Parenteral:* Intravenous amphotericin B (0.5–0.8 mg/kg/day) should be administered by slow intravenous infusion over a period of approximately 6 hours. It should be administered in 5% Dextrose. The recommended conc. for intravenous infusion is 0.1 mg/cc (1 mg/10 cc).

KETOCONAZOLE
(Oral—Fungicide, Kenazol, Nizral, Phytoral Topical—Phytoral)

Description

Ketoconazole is the first imidazole derivative which has been used successfully by oral route in the treatment of systemic fungal infections such as candidiasis, vaginal candidiasis, oral thrush and cutaneous dermatophyte infections. Ketoconazole has been found to be highly active against a broad spectrum of fungi including dermatophytes, yeast, dimorphic fungi, eumycetes, actinomycetes and some phycomycetes. It is highly effective against *Candida* and *Aspergillus* species.

Mechanism of Action

At low concentration, ketoconazole produces changes in the cell-wall of the fungi, due to which the cell volume increases and there are abnormalities in cell division. At higher concentration deterioration of all sub-cellular organelles occurs and the shape of the cell is distorted as a result of reduced osmotic resistance. Ketoconazole is extensively bound to plasma proteins. In other words the imidazole group of antifungals are fungistatic at lower dose and fungicidal at higher doses. A 200 mg oral dose yields peak serum levels in the range of 2–3 mg/l, 2–3 hours after the oral dose.

Indications

Ketoconazole is highly effective orally and is a useful adjunct to systemic antifungals in deep keratitis. The earlier the treatment is started with imidazoles the better the response.

Systemic use of ketoconazole has also been found effective in *Acanthamoeba keratitis*.

Contraindications

Ketoconazole should not be used in patients with known hypersensitivity to ketoconazole or to any other antifungal imidazoles and is contraindicated in pregnancy.

Adverse Effects

When used systemically nausea and vomiting are the most common side effects of ketoconazole, incidence of which can be reduced by administration of ketoconazole with food. Alterations in liver function tests have occurred in patients on ketoconazole, these changes may be transient. In some cases, anaphylactoid reactions have been reported after first dose. Hypersensitivity reactions including urticaria and angio-edema have also been reported. Abdominal pain, urticaria pruritus and headache are the lesser common side effects.

Warning

Hepatitis has been reported with an incidence of about 1 patient per 10,000 patients. Some of these cases may represent an idiosyncratic reaction to the drug and may be unrelated to initial biochemical changes. In patients on long-term oral treatment for onychomycosis, hepatic functions should be monitored at monthly intervals.

The risk of developing hepatitis may increase in relation to duration of treatment. Therefore, before long-term treatment is administered the benefits must be weighed against possible risks. The hepatic injury caused by keto-conazole is found to be reversible upon discontinuation of therapy.

Precautions

- Absorption of ketoconazole is maximal when taken during a meal, as it depends on stomach acidity. Concomitant treatment with agents that reduce gastric secretion (anticholinergic drugs, antacids. H_2 blockers) should be avoided and, if indicated, such drugs should be taken not less than two hours after ketoconazole.
- Ketoconazole should not be co-administered with amphotericin as it induces drug resistance in the later.
- Imidazole compounds like ketoconazole may enhance the anticoagulant effect of coumarine like drugs, thus if concomitant use is envisaged the anticoagulant effect should be carefully monitored and titrated.
- Concomitant use of rifampicin with ketoconazole may reduce the blood levels of ketoconazole. This combination is therefore not recommended.
- Concomitant use of ketoconazole and phenytoin may alter the metabolism of one or both drugs.
- Concomitant use of oral ketoconazole with antiallergics like astemizole, terfanidine and cisapride should be avoided.

Dosage and Administration

- *Topical:* A 1% solution administered topically achieves relatively high concentration in the undebrided cornea.
- *Systemic:* Ketoconazole is available as 200 mg scored tablets and 100 mg per 5 ml suspension. Recommended dose is 400 mg, given once daily in single or 2 divided doses. In children above 2 years, the recommended dose is 3.3 to 6.6 mg/kg once a day.
- Duration of treatment with ketoconazole is not well defined and should be based on clinical and mycological response. Inadequate periods of treatment may yield poor response and lead to early recurrence of clinical symptoms. Minimum treatment in candidiasis is for one or two weeks.

MICONAZOLE
(Micoptic)

Description

Miconazole is a 1% sterile antifungal drug for topical application.

Clinical Pharmacology

Miconazole is an imidazole derivative with a broad spectrum of antifungal activity, Miconazole is as active as benzyl penicillin against gram-positive bacilli and cocci. A daily oral dose of 0.3 g has been well tolerated for several weeks with beneficial effects on cutaneous fungal infection. In severe infections it can be given intravenously.

Indications

Miconazole is indicated for the treatment of fungal infections of the eye including mycotic keratitis caused by susceptible organisms. It is a drug of choice in *Candida* and *Aspergillus* organisms. Can be used for *Acanthamoeba keratitis*.

Adverse Reactions

Miconazole is contraindicated in individuals with hypersensitivity to any of its components. Conjunctival chemosis and allergic reactions may be seen in some individuals.

Dosage and Administration

The initial dosage in fungal keratitis is one drop of miconazole at hourly interval, which may be gradually reduced as with the response. The drug should be continued for 2–3 weeks.

FLUCONAZOLE
(Oral–Flucan, Flucos, Syscan, Zocon
Topical Flucan, Flucomet, Syscan, Zocon)

Description

It is the first of a new subclass of synthetic triazole antifungals.

Mechanism of Action

Same as Ketoconazole.

Indications

An important role is its use in the treatment of candida endophthalmitis. Compared to other antifungals it has deeper corneal penetration.

Adverse Reactions

Systemic: When used systemically it can cause nausea, headache and skin rash.

Contraindications

Patients with liver dysfunction, pregnant and lactating women and children < 4 weeks of age.

Dosage and Administration

- *Topical:* 0.3% eye drops 4–5 times/day in mycotic keratitis.
- *For systemic use (oral or intravenous):* 100–200 mg daily in single or two divided doses. Maximum daily dose should not exceed 400 mg/day.
- Intravitreal dose is 25 micrograms in 0.1 ml.

ECONAZOLE
(Spectazole)

Description

It is an antifungal of deschloro phenethyl imidazole group.

Mechanism of Action

Is similar to that of other imidazoles.

Indications

It has greater action against filamentous fungi than yeasts.

Dosage and Administration

It is dispensed as a 2% solution.
Oral dose: 200 mg/three times a day.

ITRACONAZOLE
(Oral—Canditral, Itaspor;
Topical—Itral drops and ointment)

Description

It has a newer triazole that has improved action against filamentous fungi. However, its poor water solubility makes it less attractive than fluconazole. It is available as a suspension, to be shaken before use.

Indications

It was found effective in 70% of keratomycosis when used orally or topically or in combination.

Adverse Effects

Gastrointestinal disturbances, headache, reversible hepatitis.

Dose

- *Oral:* 200 mg–400 mg/day in single or 2 divided doses
- *Topical:* Available as 1% eyedrops.

CASPOFUNGIN ACETATE
(Cancidas)

Description

50 mg and 70 mg vials of caspofungin are available for intravenous use.

Pharmacology

Caspofungin is an antifungal of echinocandin group derived from Glaria lozovensis. Its antifungal activity is because of inhibition of the fungal enzyme $\beta(1, 3)$-D-glucan synthase thus leading to deficient cell wall synthesis.

Indications and Usage

It is effective against *Candida* and *Aspergillus* species. It is indicated for serious fungal infections by these species when there is intolerance or lack of response to other antifungal drugs. It has been used successfully in invasive fungal endophthalmitis.

Precautions

Patients with already impaired hepatic function should be monitored for hepatic status. Concomitant use of cyclosporine should be avoided. Vials should be stored at 2° to 8°C. Reconstituted medication can be kept for one hour at ≤ 25°C and should not be infused in dextrose solutions. Final diluted solution in NaCl or Ringers lactate can be stored at ≤ 25°C for 24 hours or at 2 to 8°C for 48 hours.

Adverse Reactions

Nausea, vomiting, diarrhoea, headache, fever, hypokalemia and altered hepatic function have been associated with caspofungin therapy. Infusion related hypersensitive reactions can occur.

Dosage and Administration

Usually 50 mg once daily dose is recommended for 14 days after 70 mg loading dose on first day. It is administered by slow IV infusion over one hour. The duration of treatment is to be judged by the response and progress of improvement.

VORICONAZOLE
(Voritrol, Vfend)

Description

It is an antifungal drug available as 200 mg vial, 50 mg tablet, 200 mg tablet, and 100 ml suspension.

Pharmacology

It is a triazole drug with efficacy against *Candida*, *Aspergillus*, *Fusarium* and *Scedosporium* fungi. It acts by inhibiting ergosterol synthesis in the fungal cell wall.

Indications and Usage

Indicated for serious multidrug resistant fungal infections. It is used to treat candidemia, invasive aspergillosis and infections by *Fusarium* and *Scedosporium* spp. It has also been used to treat serious corneal fungal infections.

Adverse Reactions

Visual disturbances related to acuity, field and colour have been reported. Hepatic dysfunction is to be monitored. Other side effects are fever, rash, vomiting, nausea, diarrhea, headache, sepsis, peripheral edema, abdominal pain, and respiratory disorder. Infusion related side effects can occur.

Contraindications

Pregnancy and patients with the hereditary problem of galactose intolerance.

Dosage and Administration

IV dose is 6 mg/kg every 12 hours for the first 24 hours then 4 mg/kg 12 hourly for 14 days. Reconstituted drug should be diluted to 5 mg/ml or less and infused at a maximum rate of 3 mg/kg over one to two hours. Tablets and oral suspension should be taken one hour before or after meals.

ANIDULÁFUNGIN
(Eraxis)

Description

Anidulafungin is an antifungal drug available as 50 mg, 100 mg and 200 mg vials for intravenous infusion.

Pharmacology

Anidulafungi belongs to the echinocandin class of antifungal drugs. It acts against *Candida* by inhibiting the enzyme glucan synthase which is essential for fungal cell wall synthesis.

Indications and Usage

It is recommended for use in severe candida infections.

Adverse Reactions

Diarrhoea, hypersensitivity reactions and hepatic dysfunction may occur.

Contraindications

Contraindicated in persons with known hypersensitivity to anidulafungin or other echinocandins.

Dosage and Administration

Reconstituted vials should be added to 5% dextrose or 0.9% NaCl solution to make an infusion of concentration 0.43 mg/ml (50 mg vial) or 0.36 mg/ml (100/200 mg vial). Rate of infusion should not exceed 1.1 mg/minute. 200 mg should be given as loading dose on the first day followed by 100 mg daily for 14 days.

MICAFUNGIN
(Mycamine)

Description

Micafungin is a member of the echinocandin class of antifungal drug. It is a sterile, lyophilized product for intravenous (IV) infusion that contains micafungin sodium.

Each single-use vial contains 50 mg or 100 mg micafungin sodium.

Pharmacology

Micafungin sodium is a semisynthetic lipopeptide (echinocandin) synthesized by a chemical modification of a fermentation product of Coleophoma empetri F-11899. Micafungin inhibits the synthesis of 1, 3-β-D-glucan, an integral component of the fungal cell wall.

Indications and Usage

Indicated for serious candida infections. Efficacy for fungi other than *Candida* is not established.

Adverse Reactions

Diarrhea, nausea, vomiting, pyrexia, hypokalemia, thrombocytopenia, and headache have been reported. Hypersensitivity reactions, renal and hepatic impairment and hematological adverse effects may occur.

Dosage and Administration

Mycamine must be diluted with 0.9% sodium chloride injection, or 5% Dextrose injection. Mycamine should be administered by intravenous infusion only; 100 mg has to be infused over one hour once daily.

POSACONAZOLE
(Noxafil)

Description

Available as oral suspension containing 40 mg/ml of posaconazole.

Pharmacology

Posaconazole inhibits lanosterol 14 alpha-demethylase, the enzyme important for synthesis of the fungal cell wall component-ergosterol.

Indications and Usage

Indicated for invasive *Aspergillus* and severe *Candida* indictions unresponsive to itraconazole or fluconazole. It is also effective against *Zygomycetes* spp.

Dosage and Administration

It is given 600–800 mg/day in divided doses.

Adverse Reactions

The most common adverse effects reported are nausea and headache. Rash, dry skin, nausea, taste disturbance, abdominal pain, dizziness and flushing can also occur. Posaconazole can cause liver dysfunction in some patients.

SILVER SULFADIAZINE
(SSZ Applicap)

Description

Silver sulfadiazine 1% w/v is a sterile preparation for topical use. It is a combination of silver ions with sulfadiazine.

Mechanism of Action

Silver sulfadiazine has a broad spectrum and activity and synergistic advantage of the combination of silver ions with antibacterial activity of sulfadiazine. It has a powerful antibacterial activity and fungistatic activity against a large number of organisms. It has been suggested that combination of silver with sulfa drugs functions as an organic base-heavy metal release system. The release of silver ions is responsible for its antimicrobial action.

Indications and Usage

For the treatment of *Aspergillus, Candida, Fusarium* and dematiaceous induced mycotic keratitis. It is effective in superficial and deep mycotic keratitis.

Contraindications

Silver sulfadiazine is contraindicated in individuals who are hypersensitive to any components of the drug.

Dosage and Administration

The initial preferred dosage is one drop every hourly in the first week. The frequency may be reduced gradually with the response. Therapy should be continued for 2–4 weeks depending upon the ulcer healing.

ANTIPARASITIC AGENTS

PROPAMIDINE ISETHIONATE
(Brolene)

Description

Belongs to the diamidine group and is available as Brolene eyedrops that are available as a 0.1% solution with a preservative that is mainly paraban.

Mechanism of Action

Inhibition of DNA synthesis.

Indications and Usage

Used for *Acanthamoeba keratitis*. Published reports indicate it to be very effective. It is amebicidal and cysticidal.

Side Effects

Local irritation and superficial necrosis of granulation tissue has been observed after topical application to the wounded cornea for >10 days.

Dosage and Administration

One drop every 30 minutes for 3 days. Maintenance therapy is 1 drop every 4 hours for 3–4 weeks.

POLYHEXAMETHYLENE BIGUANIDE (PHMB)

Description

It belongs to the biguanide group which has potent antimicrobial activity. It has been used as a contact lens disinfectant in lower concentration. It is available as 0.02% solution.

Mechanism of Action

It is a cationic antiseptic.

Indications and Usage

PHMB is known to cure *Acanthamoeba keratitis* when other agents have failed.

Side Effects

Local: No corneal side effects are known.

Dosage and Administration

One drop every hour for 3 days followed by maintenance therapy.

ALBENDAZOLE
(Albendol, Alminth, Nowarm, Zentel)

Description

It is a benzaimidazole with broad spectrum antihelminthic activity.

Mechanism of Action

Inhibition of microtubule polymerization.

Indications and Usage

It is the drug of choice for cysticercus. It has been also used for treatment of retinal toxocariasis.

Side Effects

Systemic: Headache, dizziness, gastrointestinal upset.

Contraindication

Contraindicated in pregnancy due to its teratogenic potential. It should not be used for intraocular cysticercus.

Dosage and Administration

Oral dose in extraocular cysticercus is 15 mg/kg body weight/day for 30 days. Its gastrointestinal absorption is increased if it is given with a fatty meal.

4

Steroidal Antiinflammatory Agents

Common Ophthalmic Indications for Steroids

Anterior Segment (Topical)

- Allergic keratoconjunctivitis
- Interstitial keratitis
- Marginal corneal ulcer
- Chemical/electrical injury to cornea
- Immune graft rejection
- Scleritis, episcleritis
- Iritis, irido cyclitis.

Posterior Segment (Injectable, Systemic)

- Sympathetic ophthalmia
- Posterior uveitis
- Vasculitis
- Optic neuritis.

Others

- Thyroid ophthalmopathy
- Temporal arteritis
- Pseudotumor.

Mechanism of Action of Corticosteroids

Corticosteroids act as antiinflammatory drugs by inhibiting the processes involved at the site of tissue injury such as edema, deposition of fibrin, vasodilation, leukocyte migration, capillary and fibroblast proliferation, deposition of collagen and scar formation. The exact mechanism of action of corticosteroids is not very clear but most probably it is due to induction of lipocortins by the corticosteroids. These lipocortins inhibit phospholipase A2. Phospholipase A2 leads to the production of arachidonic acid from inflamed cells which further stimulates the production of prostaglandins and leukotrienes, the mediators responsible for various inflammatory changes. Thus the lipocortins induced by steroids help in controlling inflammation.

After topical application some systemic absorption does take place but that is not significant enough to produce any untoward effect.

Steroid Therapy Regimen

A steroid preparation is selected based on its potency and the prevailing severity of inflammation. The treatment should not continue for extended periods and should not be for more than three weeks in external inflammatory conditions of the eye. With signs of improvement, the dosage is reduced (tapered) from four times daily to two times and then once daily. Unless there is any serious adverse reaction, generally steroid therapy should not be stopped abruptly.

BETAMETHASONE SODIUM PHOSPHATE
(Betnesol, Betnesol- N, Betnor, Garasone)

Description

Betamethasone 0.1% ointment and drops have topical antiinflammatory activity.

Contraindications

In viral, fungal infections or tuberculosis use is contra-indicated. Also if patient has glaucoma or has a family history of glaucoma the use of steroids should be avoided.

It is contraindicated in persons showing hypersensitivity to any component of the preparation.

Side Effects

- *Local:* Steroid induced glaucoma can cause rise in intraocular pressure in a small percentage of the population especially those with a family history of glaucoma.
- Thinning of the cornea leading to perforation has occurred with the use of topical corticosteroids.
- Cataract may occur after prolonged use.
- Delayed wound healing
- Ptosis
- *Systemic:* It should be noted that 0.1% betamethasone four times a day in each eye is equivalent to 0.25 mg of oral betamethasone. Hence depending on the dose the systemic side effects of steroids may occur after local use.

Dosage and Administration

1–2 drops instilled into the eye every one or two hours until control of inflammation is achieved, after which the frequency may be reduced.

DEXAMETHASONE SODIUM PHOSPHATE
(Dexcin, Dexamet-N,Decol-C, Dexoren S)

Description

Dexamethasone sodium phosphate is a water-soluble form of the synthetic antiinflammatory steroid dexamethasone. Available as 0.05–0.1% ophthalmic solution and 0.5% ointment usually available in combination with antibacterials.

Actions

It causes inhibition of inflammatory response to inciting agents of mechanical, chemical or immunological nature.

Contraindications

- Acute herpes simplex keratitis.
- Fungal corneal ulcer.
- Vaccinia, varicella and most other viral diseases of the cornea and conjunctiva.
- Hypersensitivity to a component of this medication.

Warnings

- Steroid medication in the treatment of herpes simplex keratitis involving the stroma requires great caution, frequent slit lamp microscopy is mandatory.
- Prolonged use may result in glaucoma, which may be especially common among children.
- Posterior subcapsular cataract formation
- May aid in the establishment of secondary ocular infection from pathogens liberated from ocular tissues.
- *Usage in pregnancy:* Safety of intensive or protracted use of topical steroids during pregnancy has not been established.

Precautions

As fungal/viral infection of the cornea are particularly prone to develop coincidentally with long-term steroid applications, these must be suspected in any persistent corneal ulceration where a steroid has been used or is in use. Intraocular pressure should be checked frequently.

Adverse Reactions

Glaucoma, posterior subcapsular cataract formation, secondary ocular infection from pathogens liberated from ocular tissues like viral keratitis.

On intravenous use of dexamethasone, patient can have utricaria/rash or erythema.

Dosage and Administration

- *Initially:* 1–2 drops placed in the conjunctival sac every hour until improvement occurs. Thereafter gradually reduce to 1–2 drops every 3 or 4 hours.
- *Ointment:* Apply a thin coating of ointment three or four times a day, when a favorable response is observed, reduce the number of daily applications to two, and later to once a day as a maintenance dose if this is sufficient to control symptoms.
- *Intravitreal:* 400 µg/0.1ml
- *Pulse therapy:* Dexamethasone 200 mg in 150 ml of 5% dextrose over 1 hour.

PREDNISOLONE
(P-lone, Predmet, Predaccetate)

Description

Prednisolone acetate 1% is a synthetic corticosteroid. Prednisolone acetate is available as 1% suspension. In comparison, prednisolone phophate is a solution. Also available in combination with chloramphenicol 0.2%, sulfacetamide sodium 10% and neomycin HCl. It has 3 to 5 times the antiinflammatory potency of hydrocortisone. Like all glucocorticoids it inhibits edema, fibrin deposition, capillary dilatation and phagocytic migration of the acute inflammatory response as well as capillary proliferation, deposition of collagen and scar formation.

Contraindications

Acute untreated purulent ocular infections, acute superficial herpes simplex (dendritic keratitits) vaccinia, varicella and most other viral diseases of the cornea and conjunctiva, fungal diseases of the eye and sensitivity to any components of the formulation.

Adverse Reactions

Steroid induced ocular hypertension, glaucoma, posterior subcapsular cataract formation, secondary ocular infections from fungi or viruses liberated from ocular tissues and perforation of the globe when used in conditions where there is thinning of the cornea or sclera.

Dosage and Administration

1–2 drops instilled into the conjunctival sac two to four times daily. During the initial 24 to 48 hours the dosage may be safely increased to 2 drops every hour. Care should be taken not to discontinue therapy prematurely.

METHYLPREDNISOLONE
(Solu-Medrol, Depo-Medrol)

Description

Methylprednisolone is available as a shorter acting preparation called methylprednisolone sodium succinate and a longer acting methylprednisolone acetate.

Adverse Reactions

Similar as for other steroids.

Contraindications

Periocular injections are contraindicated in toxoplasmosis and necrotising scleritis.

Dosage and Administration

- *Local:* Methylprednisolone sodium succinate is administered as a periocular injection of 40 mg/ml or 125 mg/2 ml. It is water soluble and diffuses rapidly from the depot. In contrast methylprednisolone acetate is administered as 40–80 mg/0.5 ml and is longer acting.
- *Systemic:* Methylprednisolone sodium succinate is used for pulse therapy as 1 gm/day for 3 days for optic neuritis.

TRIAMCINOLONE ACETONIDE
(Inj-Kenocort, Ledercort, Pericort 4, Tricort)

Description

Compared to other steroids triamcinolone has no mineralo-corticoid activity.

Indications

Periocular triamcinolone is preferred as it has lesser tendency to cause scar formation and extraocular muscle fibrosis. The treatment effect after periocular injection is apparent after 2–3 days. Injections can be repeated after 2–4 weeks as dictated by the clinician. Effect of intravitreal injections lasts for 6–9 months. It has been used as intravitreal implants.

Contraindications

Periocular injections are contraindicated in toxoplasmosis and necrotising scleritis.

Precautions

When injected in the peribulbar/retrobulbar space it has the harmful potential of causing extraocular muscle fibrosis especially if the injection is given by mistake in the muscle belly.

Dosage and Administration

- *Periocular:* 20–40 mg subconjunctival/subtenon injections.
- Intravitreal triamcinolone injection of 4–25 mg can be administered after passing the suspension through a millipore filter for at least 3 times so as to get a clear solution. For age-related macular degeneration 4 mg/0.1 ml can be given, while higher dose may be required for macular edema associated with diabetic retinopathy or CRVO.

HYDROCORTISONE ACETATE
(Efcorlin)

Warnings

Prolonged use may result in elevated intraocular pressure and may cause glaucomatous damage to the optic nerve, defects in visual acuity and fields of vision, posterior subcapsular cataract formation or may result in secondary ocular infections. Viral, fungal and bacterial infections of the eye may be exacerbated by the application of steroids. Acute purulent untreated infection of the eye or ear may be masked or activity enhanced by the presence of steroid medication. In those diseases causing thinning of the cornea or sclera, perforation has been known to occur with the use of topical steroids.

As fungal infections of the cornea are particularly prone to develop coincidentally with long-term local steroid applications, fungus may be considered in any persistent corneal ulceration where a steroid has been used or is in use.

Dosage and Administration

The duration of treatment will vary with the type of lesion and may extend from a few days to several weeks according to the therapeutic response. Instill one or two drops into the conjunctival sac every hour during the day and every two hours during the night as initial therapy. When a favorable response is observed, reduce dosage to one drop every four hours.

MEDRYSONE
(HMS liquifilm)

Description

Medrysone 1% drops belongs to the family of steroids, related structurally more to progesterone than to other available corticosteroids. It is available as a suspension.

Medrysone is a synthetic steroid with topical antiinflammatory and antiallergic activity. Medrysone has less antiinflammatory potency than 0.1% dexamethasone. In patients with increased intraocular pressure and in those susceptible to a rise in intraocular pressure, there is less effect on pressure with medrysone than with dexamethasone or betamethasone.

Contraindications

Medrysone is contraindicated in the following conditions: Acute superficial herpes simplex viral diseases of the conjunctiva and cornea, ocular tuberculosis and fungal diseases of the eye.

Warnings

Similar as for other steroids.

Adverse Reactions

Occasional transient stinging and burning may occur on instillation.

Dosage and Administration

One drop instilled in the conjunctival sac up to every four hours. Shake well before using.

Relative Potency of Commonly used Oral Steroids

Drug	Oral dose (mg)
Betamethasone	3
Dexamethasone	3
Triamcinolone	12
Methylprednisolone	15
Prednisolone	15
Hydrocortisone	60

FLUOROMETHOLONE
(Flosef, FML forte)

Description

It is metabolized in the cornea.

Indications

It is primarily used in mild anterior segment inflammation and post-LASIK surgery.

Dosage and Administration

It is available as a suspension in 5 ml vials in 0.1% strength and in 0.25% (FML forte). One drop is to be administered two to four times daily.

RIMEXOLONE
(Pom-vexol)

Description

It is available as 1% suspension. Each ml contains rimexolone 10 mg and 0.01% benzalkonium chloride preservative. It is more potent a steroid than fluromethalone.

Indications

Anterior segment inflammation, especially that following cataract surgery. Its efficacy is similar to 1% prednisolone acetate.

Adverse Reactions

Ocular: Occur in 1–5% patients and include blurred vision, ocular pain, increased IOP, foreign body sensation and corneal ulcer.

Contraindications

Epithelial herpes simplex keratitis and most other viral diseases of the cornea and conjunctiva. Fungal disease of the eye and acute purulent untreated infections which may be masked or enhanced by the presence of steroids.

Dosage and Administration

In anterior uveitis every hour for the first week and then to be tapered. After surgery one drop 4 times/day for 2 weeks. The vial should be shaken well before use.

LOTEPREDNOL ETABONATE
(Alrex, Lotemax, Lpred)

Description

It is a steroid preparation with powerful antiinflammatory activity and low propensity to increase IOP. It has high lipophilicity with good intraocular penetration.

Indications

It is being primarily used for post-LASIK surgery inflammation. It can also be used in seasonal allergic conjunctivitis.

Contraindications

Similar to rimexolone.

Dosage and Administration

It is available as a 0.2% and 0.5% ophthalmic suspension. One drop to be instilled four times daily in affected eye(s).

DIFLUPREDNATE
(Durezo, Duronet)

Description

Is a topical antiinflammatory steroid available as 0.05% ophthalmic emulsion. Its long half-life supports less frequent dosage. It does not contain BAK preservative but has sorbic acid as a preservative.

Indications and Usage

Recommended to treat pain and inflammation associated with ocular surgery.

Dosage and Administration

One drop four times daily is to be instilled in the conjunctival sac beginning 24 hours postoperatively for two weeks followed by one drop two times daily for one week and then tapered depending on the response.

Adverse Reactions

Adverse reactions include corneal edema, ciliary and conjunctival hyperemia, eye pain, photophobia, posterior capsule opacification, anterior chamber cells, anterior chamber fare, conjunctival edema, and blepharitis. Reduced visual acuity, punctate keratitis, eye infammation, and iritis can also be seen. Application site discomfort or irritation, corneal pigmentation and striae, episcleritis, eye pruritis, eyelid irritation and crusting, foreign body sensation, increased lacrimation, macular edema, scleral hyperemia, and uveitis are less common. More so these symptoms and signs could result from the surgical procedure itself.

As with other steroids there is an associated risk of increased intraocular pressure, posterior subcapsular cataract, secondary infections and perforation of globe.

Precautions

Contraindicated in most active viral diseases of the cornea and conjunctiva including epithelial herpes simplex keratitis (dendritic keratitis), vaccinia, and varicella, and also in mycobacterial and fungal infections.

Topical Nonsteroidal Antiinflammatory and Antiallergic Agents

5

MECHANISM OF ACTION OF NSAIDs

NSAIDs afford relief in inflammatory conditions but do not modify the underlying pathology. The inflammation mainly occurs due to the release or synthesis of chemical mediator, which include histamine, kinins, prostaglandins (PGs) and the platelet-activating factor. These mediators interact amongst each other and potentiate the biological effects.

Roles of prostaglandins have been extensively studied in inflammation. It is now well established that NSAIDs inhibit the formation and synthesis of PGs that has been suggested to be the mechanisms of action of most NSAIDs.

The synthesis of PGs is dependent upon the activity of enzyme cyclo-oxygenase, while formation of leukotrienes is dependent upon the activity of lipo-oxygenase. Leukotrienes influence leukocyte response to inflammation and have been suggested to cause aggregation of polymorpho nuclear (PMN) leukocytes as well as chemotaxis and chemokinesis. Most of the NSAIDs inhibit enzyme cyclo-oxygenase whereas some of them inhibit both cyclo-oxygenase and lipo-oxygenase. Thus those NSAIDs which block both the enzymes are likely to be more effective antiinflammatory drugs.

Common Adverse Effects of Topical NSAIDs

All topical nonsteroidal antiinflammatory drugs (NSAIDs), have the potential of delaying wound healing. The risk may further increase if they are used concomitantly with topical steroids.

Keratitis, epithelial breakdown, corneal thinning, corneal erosion, corneal ulceration or corneal perforation may occur in susceptible patients on prolonged use of topical NSAIDs. So these should be used with caution in patients with complicated or repeat ocular surgeries, corneal denervation, corneal epithelial defects, diabetes mellitus, ocular surface diseases and rheumatoid arthritis.

INDOMETHACIN
(Indoflam)

Description

Indomethacin is a colourless solution 1% w/v with thiomersal as preservative and buffered with boric acid and sodium hydroxide to adjust the pH to 7.4.

Indications and Usage

For the treatment of inflammatory conditions of the conjunctiva, cornea, allergic conjunctivitis, superficial punctate keratitis, iritis, cystoid macular edema and allergic conjunctivitis.

Mechanism of Action

Indomethacin is one of the most potent inhibitors of prostaglandin forming cyclo-oxygenase. It inhibits motility of polymorphonuclear leukocytes. It may also inhibit the proliferation of B-cells and T-cells. It can inhibit phospholipase A and C. Like many other aspirin like drugs indomethacin uncouples oxidative phosphorylation in supratherapeutic concentrations and depresses the biosynthesis of mucopolysaccharides.

Contraindications

Known hypersensitivity to thiomersal. If irritation persists or increases, discontinue use and consult the physician.

Dosage and Administration

1–2 drops in affected eye four times a day. It should be stored in a cool place and protected from sunlight.

FLURBIPROFEN SODIUM
(Ocuflur, FBN)

Description

Flurbiprofen sodium 0.03% is an antiinflammatory product for topical ophthalmic use.

Clinical Pharmacology

Flurbiprofen sodium is one of a series of phenyl alkonoic acids that have shown analgesic, antipyretic and antiinflammatory activity in inflammatory diseases. It acts through inhibition of the cyclo-oxygenase enzyme that is essential in the bio-synthesis of prostaglandins.

Indications and Usage

Flurbiprofen is indicated for the inhibition of intra-operative miosis. It can also be used to treat post-laser and post-operative anterior segment inflammation of eye.

Contraindications

Flurbiprofen is contraindicated in epithelial herpes simplex keratitis (dendritic keratitis) and in individuals who are hypersensitive to any components of the medication.

Warnings

There exists the potential for cross-sensitivity to acetyl salicylic acid and other non-steroidal antiinflammatory drugs. Therefore, caution should be used when treating individuals who have previously exhibited sensitivities to these drugs.

Adverse Reactions

Transient burning and stinging upon instillation has been reported. It is recommended that flurbiprofen be used with caution in patients with bleeding tendencies as it may increase the bleeding time by interference with thrombocyte aggregation.

Dosage and Administration

A total of four drops of flurbiprofen should be administered by instilling 1 drop approximately every 30 min, beginning 2 hours before surgery to prevent intraoperative miosis.

DICLOFENAC SODIUM
(Oxalgin, Voveran ophtha)

Description

Diclofenac sodium is available as 0.1% solution.

Pharmacology

Diclofenac sodium is a potent non-steroidal anti-inflammatory drug with analgesic activity, which inhibits prostaglandin synthesis.

Indications and Usage

Postoperative inflammation after cataract extraction, macular edema, prevention of surgically induced miosis, non-infectious inflammatory conditions in the eye, and post-traumatic inflammation as an adjunct to antimicrobial therapy. It is also used to temporarily relieve eye pain and sensitivity to light in patients who are recovering from corneal refractive surgery.

Contraindications

Hypersensitivity to NSAIDs, those wearing contact lenses and during surgical procedures.

Adverse Reactions

Transient burning sensation, photosensitivity, ocular allergy, delayed healing and rarely keratitis. Severe corneal melting was reported when diclofenac was used with a solubilizer called tocophersolan. Diclofenac reduces a neuropeptide called substance P in human tears. This may induce conditions conducive to the development of neurotrophic keratopathy.

Dosage and Administration

Drops: 1–2 drops 3–4 times daily.

For ocular surgery 1 drop every hour preoperatively beginning 3 hours before. Continue postoperatively 1 drop thrice a day, throughout the first 2 weeks of the postoperative period.

SUPROFEN
(Suprol)

Description

Suprofen is available as 1% topical ophthalmic solution.

Pharmacology

Following topical application it achieves significant intraocular levels and inhibits the release of prostaglandin E2 and F2a and thromboxane B_2 from the inflamed cornea more effectively.

Indications and Usage

It is a good NSAID in treating giant papillary conjunctivitis, iatrogenic inflammation of the eye and in preventing intraoperative miosis.

Adverse Effects

Eye burning, stinging, irritation, itching, redness, or sensitivity to light.

Contraindications

It is contraindicated in epithelial herpes simplex keratitis (dendritic keratitis) and in those with known hypersensitivity to suprofen.

Dosage and Administration

To put 2 drops at 1, 2, 3 hours preoperatively to prevent intraoperative miosis and four times a day postoperatively for any postoperative inflammation.

KETOROLAC TROMETHAMINE
(Ketanov, Keflur, Acular)

Description

Ketorolac tromethamine is available as 0.5% solution.

Indications and Usage

Indicated for relief of ocular itching due to seasonal allergic conjunctivitis. Also used in post excimer surgery, pain management, chronic conjunctivitis and iatrogenic inflammation of the eye and sometimes for topical treatment of cystoid macular edema.

Adverse Reactions

Transient stinging and burning sensation on instillation. Other ocular adverse effects reported are ocular irritation, allergic reactions, superficial ocular irritation and rarely superficial keratitis.

Caution

Should be used with caution in patients with known bleeding tendencies or who are receiving other medications, which may prolong bleeding time.

Dosage and Administration

The recommended dose is one drop four times a day. It should not be used in patients wearing soft contact lenses.

BROMFENAC
(Bromifen, BFN, Megabrom)

Description

Bromfenac is a topical, nonsteroidal antiinflammatory drug (NSAID) for ophthalmic use formulated as 0.09% solution.

Pharmacology

It blocks prostaglandin synthesis by inhibiting cyclo-oxygenase 1 and 2, thus acting as antiinflammatory drug.

Indications and Usage

It is indicated for the treatment of postoperative inflammation in patients who have undergone cataract extraction.

Dosage and Administration

One drop of bromfenac solution should be applied to the affected eye(s) two times daily beginning 24 hours after cataract surgery and continuing through the first 2 weeks of the postoperative period.

Adverse Reactions

Abnormal sensation in eye, burning/stinging sensation, pain, pruritus, redness, headache, and iritis and keratitis may be associated or can also occur due to surgery itself.

Precaution

There is an increased risk of bleeding, delayed corneal healing if used with concomitant topical steroids. Continued use for more than 24 hours before surgery and after 14 days of surgery predisposes to keratitis and corneal adverse reactions. Rarely systemic side effects like exacerbation of asthma and gastrointestinal bleeding have been reported with topical use of NSAIDS.

NEPAFENAC
(Nepaflam, Nepalact, Nevanac)

Description

Nepafenac 0.1% is available for use as antiinflammatory topical ophthalmic suspension. Unlike other topical NSAIDS nepafenac is not a free acid.

Mechanism of Action

After topical ocular application, nepafenac penetrates the cornea and is converted to Amfenac. Amfenac has nonsteroidal antiinflammatory action. It inhibits the synthesis of prostaglandins, which are responsible for pain and inflammation, by inhibiting the enzyme cyclooxygenase (prostaglandin synthase). Following topical application its effect begins in 15 minutes and duration of action lasts at least 8 hours.

Indications and Usage

It is indicated for the treatment of pain and inflammation associated with cataract and refractive surgery. When applied topically it achieves higher aqueous concentrations compared to bromfenac and ketorolac.

Adverse Reactions

Adverse effects that may be associated with nepafenac use are–capsular opacity, decreased visual acuity, foreign body sensation, puntacte keratopathy, and sticky sensation.

Precautions

Increased bleeding time and keratitis have been reported. Hypersensitivity to any of the ingredients in the formulation or to other NSAIDs is a contraindication for use. It should be used with caution in nursing mothers.

Dosage and Administration

One drop is to be instilled in the affected eye(s) three-times-daily starting on the day before surgery and then continued up to the first 2 weeks of the postoperative period.

ANTIALLERGICS

Most of the clinical symptoms of allergy including vasodilation and the edema of conjunctiva and eyelid margins are mainly because of the effects of histamine. In cases of allergy the main aim should be to recognize the offending allergen, avoiding/removing such factor, maintenance of proper tear film and carefully selecting drugs according to the type of allergy and expected duration of therapy. General measures such as cold compress and washing the eyes also help in improving the symptoms.

The symptoms of seasonal, vernal and several types of papillary conjunctivitis do not subside by the general measures and use of decongestants or histamine receptor blocking agents only. They do not have preventive effect against the release of new histamine. But the reduction in the total histamine secretion is as important for chronic cases of allergic conjunctivitis and needs the intervention by mast cell stabilizers. In severe chronic cases with prominent symptoms, a combination therapy of antihistamines, mast cell stabilizers and decongestants may be necessary.

SODIUM CROMOGLYCATE
(Fintal, Cromal)

Description

Sodium cromoglycate is a clear colorless 4% solution. In vitro and in vivo studies have shown that sodium cromoglycate inhibits the degranulation of sensitized mast cells which occurs after exposure to specific antigens. Sodium cromoglycate inhibits the release of histamine and SRS-A. Bronchial asthma induced by the inhalation of specific antigens can be inhibited to varying degree by pretreatment with sodium cromoglycate. Another activity demonstrated in vitro is the capacity of sodium cromoglycate to inhibit the degranulation of non-sensitized mast cells by phospholipase-A and the subsequent release of chemical mediators.

Indications and Usage

For the treatment of vernal keratoconjunctivitis, chronic allergic conjunctivitis and acute allergic conjunctivitis such as hay fever.

Contraindications

Known hypersensitivity to sodium cromoglycate.

Precautions

Store in a cool place. Protect from direct sunlight. Discard any remaining contents four weeks after opening the bottle. If irritation persists or increases discontinue the use and consult physician. Do not touch the dropper tip or other dispensing tip to any surface since this may contaminate the solution.

Dosage and Administration

One or two drops into each eye four times daily.

NEDOCROMIL SODIUM
(Alocril)

Description

It is a mast cell stabilizer that inhibits the release of mediators from cells involved in hypersensitivity reactions. It is available as a 2% solution.

Indications

Allergic conjunctivitis.

Adverse reactions

Headache is the most common side effect. Others include ocular burning, stinging and irritation.

Warning

Do not use while wearing contact lenses.

Dosage

1–2 drops twice a day. Treatment should be continued till the exposure to the allergen is terminated.

LODOXAMIDE TROMETHAMINE
(Lomide)

Description

It is a mast cell stabilizer that inhibits type 1 hypersensitivity reaction, dispensed as a 0.1% solution. It is 250 times more potent than cromolyn sodium.

Indications

Vernal keratoconjunctivitis, superior limbic keratoconjunctivitis.

Adverse Reactions

Local: Transient burning, stinging sensation
Systemic: Headache, heat sensation, somnolence.

Warning

As with all ophthalmic preparations containing benzalkonium chloride, instruct patient not to wear contact lens during treatment with lodoxamide.

Dosage

1–2 drops, 4 times a day.

OLOPATADINE HCL
(Patanol)

Description

It is a selective H1 receptor antagonist that inhibits type 1 hypersensitivity reaction and is dispensed as a 0.1% solution. It has a rapid onset of action that lasts 8 hours.

Indications

Allergic conjunctivitis.

Adverse Reactions

Local: Burning, stinging, FB sensation
Systemic: Headache.

Warning

Contact lens wearers.

Dosage

1–2 drops 2 times/day.

KETOTIFEN FUMARATE
(Albalon, Ketorid)

Description

This antiallergic is available as 0.025% ophthalmic solution.

Pharmacology

Ketotifen is a relatively selective, non-competitive histamine (H1)-receptor antagonist and mast cell stabilizer. It has also been found to decrease activation of eosinophils and chemotaxis. It is claimed to act fast (within minutes).

Indications and Usage

It is indicated for relief of itching due to allergic conjunctivitis.

Dosage and Administration

1 drop in the affected eye(s) to be instilled twice daily, every 8–12 hours (no more than twice per day).

Adverse Reactions

Mild side effects such as conjunctival injection, headaches, and rhinitis have been reported. Less commonly, allergic reactions, flu syndrome, and pharyngitis may occur.

AZELASTINE HYDROCHLORIDE
(Azelast, Oculast)

Description

Azelastine is an antiallergic drug available for use as 0.05% solution for topical administration.

Pharmacology

It is a relatively selective histamine(H1) antagonist and an inhibitor of the release of histamine. Inhibition of other mediators (e.g. leukotrienes and PAF) from cells involved in allergic reactions has been demonstrated with Azelastine hydrochloride. Decreased chemotaxis and activation of eosinophils has also been demonstrated. Effect is claimed to begin within minutes and lasts for 8–12 hours.

Indications and Usage

Indicated for relief of symptoms in seasonal and perennial allergic conjunctivitis.

Dosage and Administration

One drop is to be instilled in the affected eye twice daily. If necessary the dose can be increased to four times daily.

Adverse Reactions

Mild transient eye burning of eyes, headache and bitter taste may occur.

Contraindicated

Contraindicated in persons with known or suspected hypersensitivity to any of its components.

EPINASTINE HCL
(Relestat)

Description

Epinastine HCl is an antihistamine and available as 0.05% topical ophthalmic solution.

Pharmacology

Epinastine HCl is a histamine (H1) receptor antagonist and an inhibitor of histamine release from the mast cell.

Indications and Usage

It is recommended for use in the prevention of itching associated with allergic conjunctivitis.

Dosage and Administration

One drop in each eye is instilled twice a day. Treatment should be continued throughout the period of allergic risk or until exposure to the offending allergen is terminated, even when symptoms are absent.

Precautions

Contraindicated in those patients who have shown hypersensitivity to epinastine or to any of the other ingredients.

Adverse Reactions

Burning sensation in the eye, folliculosis, hyperemia, itching and flu like symptoms can occur.

BEPOTASTINE BESILATE
(Bepreve)

Description

Bepotastine besilate is available as 1.5% topical ophthalmic solution.

Pharmacology

It is a direct histamine(H1)-receptor antagonist and also inhibits the release of histamine from mast cells.

Indications and Usage

It is indicated for relief of itching associated with allergic conjunctivitis.

Precautions

It should not be used when wearing contact lenses or to treat contact lens related irritation.

Adverse Reactions

Mild taste following instillation, ocular irritation, headache, and nasopharyngitis are the occasionally reported side effects.

Dosage and Administration

One drop should be instilled in the affected eye(s) twice a day.

PEMIROLAST
(Alamast)

Description

It is an antiallergic formulated as 0.1% pemirolast potassium for topical administration to the eyes.

Pharmacology

Pemirolast potassium inhibits the allergic inflammatory mediators (e.g. histamine, leukotriene) from mast cells. In addition, pemirolast potassium inhibits the chemotaxis of eosinophils into ocular tissue and blocks the release of mediators from eosinophils. Although the precise mechanism of action is unknown, the drug has been reported to prevent calcium influx into mast cells upon antigen stimulation.

Indications and Usage

Indicated for use in allergic conjunctivitis.

Adverse Reactions

Headache, rhinitis, flulike symptoms, burning, dry eye, and foreign body sensation can occur.

Dosage and Administration

Recommended dose is one to two drops in each affected eye four times daily. Symptomatic improvement is there within a few days, but frequently requires longer treatment (up to four weeks).

LEVOCABASTINE
(Livostin)

Description

Levocabastine hydrochloride is available as 0.05% ophthalmic suspension in 2.5 ml, 5 ml, and 10 ml vials.

Pharmacology

It is a selective histamine (H1) receptor-antagonist.

Indications and Usage

It is indicated for the temporary relief of the signs and symptoms of seasonal allergic conjunctivitis.

Adverse Reactions

Mild, transient stinging/burning sensation on instillation and headache have been reported occasionally.

Contraindications

It is contraindicated in persons with known or suspected hypersensitivity to any of its components. It should not be used while soft contact lenses are being worn.

Dosage and Administration

One drop should be instilled in the affected eye(s) four times daily.

EMEDASTINE DIFUMARATE
(Emadine)

Description

Emedastine 0.05% is an antiallergic ophthalmic solution containing topical administration to the eyes.

Pharmacology

Emedastine is a relatively selective, histamine (H1) receptor antagonist.

Indications and Usage

Indicated for the temporary relief of the signs and symptoms of allergic conjunctivitis.

Adverse Reactions

Headache is the most common side effect. Abnormal dreams, asthenia, bad taste, blurred vision, burning or stinging, corneal infiltrates, corneal staining, dermatitis, discomfort, dry eye, foreign body sensation, hyperemia, keratitis, pruritus, rhinitis, sinusitis, and tearing are other less common side effects.

Contraindications

It is contraindicated in persons with known or suspected hypersensitivity to any of its components.

Dosage and Administration

One drop is to be instilled in the affected eye(s) four times daily.

6

Miotics, Mydriatics and Cycloplegics

MIOTICS

PILOCARPINE NITRATE/HYDROCHLORIDE
(Pilocar)

Description

Pilocarpine nitrate, a sterile ophthalmic solution available as 1%, 2% or 4% drops.

Pilocarpine is a direct acting para sympathominetic drug, which duplicates the muscuranic effects of acetylcholine, but has no nicotinic effect. Pilocarpine stimulates secretory glands and smooth muscles and has no effect on striated muscle. Pilocarpine is effective in the treatment of glaucoma by improving the facility of outflow. Onset of miosis occurs within 10–30 minutes and lasts for 4–8 hours following topical application.

Indications and Usage

Indicated for:

- The control of intraocular pressure in glaucoma
- Emergency relief of mydriasis in an acutely glaucoma-tous situation
- To reverse mydriasis caused by a cycloplegic agent.

Contraindications

Pilocarpine is contraindicated in persons showing hypersensitivity to any of its components.

Warnings

Pilocarpine is readily absorbed systemically on topical application. Excessive application may elicit toxicity symptoms in some individuals.

Precautions

Pilocarpine has been reported to cause retinal detachment in individuals with pre-existing retinal diseases or predisposed to retinal tears. Safety and effectiveness in children have not been established.

Adverse Reactions

Include visual blurring due to miosis and accommodative spasm, poor dark adaptation caused by the failure of the pupil to dilate in reduced illumination and conjunctival hyperemia. Miotics have been reported to cause lens opacities in susceptible individuals after prolonged use.

Dosage and Administration

- To aid in emergency miosis 1 to 2 drops of one of the higher concentrations should be used.
- The dosage and strength required to reverse mydriasis depends on the cycloplegic used.
- Pilocarpine gel for the management of glaucoma has been marketed in United States by Alcon Laboratories. It delivers pilocarpine up to 24 hours after single night time placement in the cul-de-sac.
- Ocusert system is based on non-porous membrane. A central reservoir of the drug is surrounded by polymeric membrane which allows constant delivery of the drug at a controlled rate after an initial pulse release for approximately one week. Two types of ocuserts are

available Pilo-20 and Pilo-40, which deliver 20 µg and 40 µg pilocarpine per hour respectively.

CARBACHOL

Description

Carbachol is a cholinergic prepared as a sterile topical and intracameral ophthalmic solution. Carbachol is a direct acting parasympathomimetic that is sometime used when allergy or resistance to pilocarpine develops. Unlike pilocarpine, carbachol has both nicotinic and muscuranic actions. It is available as 0.75% drops.

Clinical Pharmacology

It is a cholinergic (parasympathominetic) agent. Carbachol has a double action. It not only stimulates the motor endplate of the muscle cell, as do all cholinesters, but it also partially inhibits cholinesterase.

Indications and Usage

For lowering intraocular pressure in the treatment of glaucoma.

Contraindications

Miotics are contraindicated where constriction is undesirable such as acute iritis. It is also contraindicated in those patients showing hypersensitivity to any component of this preparation.

Warnings

For topical and intracameral use only. Not for injection. Carbachol should be used with caution in the presence of corneal abrasion to avoid excessive penetration which can produce systemic toxicity and in patients with acute cardiac failure, bronchial asthma, active peptic ulcer, hyperthyroidism, gastrointestinal spasm, urinary tract obstruction and Parkinson's disease. As with all miotics, retinal detachment has been reported when used in certain susceptible individuals.

Precautions

Avoid over dosage. The miosis usually causes difficulty in dark adaptation. Patient should be advised to exercise caution in night driving and other hazardous occupations in poor light.

Adverse Reactions

This preparation is capable of producing systemic symptoms of a cholinesterase inhibitor even when the epithelium is intact. Transient ciliary and conjunctival injection, headache and ciliary spasm with browache and temporary decrease of visual acuity due to the induced myopia may occur. Salivation, syncope, cardiac arrhythmia, gastrointestinal cramping, vomiting, asthma and diarrhoea may occur.

Dosage and Administration

Instill two drops topically in the eye(s) up to four times daily.

PHOSPHOLINE IODIDE

Description

Phospholine iodide is available in the following concentrations: 0.03%, 0.06%, 0.125%, 0.25%.

Phospholine iodide is a long-acting cholinesterase inhibitor for topical use which enhances the effect of endogenously liberated acetylcholine of iris, ciliary muscle and other parasympathetically innervated structures of the eye. It thereby causes miosis, increase in facility of aqueous humor, fall in intraocular pressure and potentiation of accommodation.

Indications

In chronic open angle glaucoma, sub-acute or chronic angle closure glaucoma after iridectomy or where surgery is refused or contraindicated.

Contraindications

- Active uveal inflammation.
- Most cases of angle closure glaucoma due to the possibility of increasing angle block.
- Hypersensitivity to the active or inactive ingredients.

Adverse Reactions

- Stinging, burning, lacrimation, lid muscle twitching conjunctival and ciliary redness, browache induced myopia with visual blurring may occur.
- Activation of latent iritis or uveitis may occur.
- Iris cysts may form and if treatment is continued may enlarge and obscure vision. This occurrence is more frequent in children.
- Prolonged use may cause conjunctival thickening, obstruction of nasolacrimal canals.
- Lens opacities, paradoxical increase in intraocular pressure.

Dosage and Administration

Early chronic glaucoma, 0.03% instilled twice a day. Refrigerated aqueous solution shows a drop in potency within 4 weeks.

MYDRIATICS

PHENYLEPHRINE HYDROCHLORIDE
(Drosyn)

Description

Phenylephrine hydrochloride (2·5% and 10%) ophthalmic solution is primarily a direct acting drug that stimulates the alpha receptors causing contraction of dilator muscles of the iris. It also causes blanching of the conjunctival vessels.

Indications

Although the mydriasis produced by 2·5% phenylephrine alone is generally not adequate for detailed examination of the retinal periphery, it is often sufficient for viewing the posterior pole. Mydriasis produced is not accompanied by cycloplegia. It is a fast-acting mydriatic.

One drop of 2.5% phenylephrine causing > 5 mmHg rise in IOP has been used as a provocative test for angle closure. It is also used to differentiate between superficial and deep conjunctival congestion.

Contraindications

- Narrow angle glaucoma
- *Hypertensive patients:* Phenylephrine is a powerful vasoconstrictor and is absorbed systemically when applied topically to the eye.
- 10% Phenylephrine is contradicted in infants.
- In eyes where corneal epithelium is denuded it may cause corneal clouding
- Persons with a known hypersensitivity to any component.

Adverse Effects

Ophthalmic: Mild stinging on initial instillation, rebound conjunctival congestion on prolonged use, and rebound miosis may occur in some elderly patients and subsequent instillation may produce less mydriasis.

Systemic: The major difficulty in using this drug is the possibility of inducing systemic hypertension, tachycardia (especially when given to infants/neonates). Headache or browache may occur. Episodes of myocardial infarction and arrhythmias in elderly patients are reported.

Stability: One other disadvantage is relatively short shelf life as once the bottle is opened phenylephrine rapidly oxidises which makes it less effective.

Dosage and Administration

Topically 1 or 2 drops into the conjunctiva of each eye for refraction, in conjunction with some cycloplegic of choice. Maximum dilation with phenylephrine alone occurs within 15–60 minutes. The pupil size returns to normal within

4–6 hours. Initial instillation of a topical anesthetic before phenylephrine prevents the stinging caused by phenylephrine and enhances pupillary dilation.

In premature infants for dilation, 2.5% phenylephrine is used in conjunction with 0.2% cyclopentolate or 0.5% tropicamide.

ATROPINE SULFATE
(Atroren-P, Atrocin)

Description

Atropine sulfate is an anticholinergic prepared as a sterile topical ophthalmic solution and ointment supplied in three strengths: 0.5%, 1% and 3.0%.

Mechanism of Action

Atropine sulfate is a naturally occurring alkaloid that acts directly on the muscarinic receptors of structure innervated by the post-ganglionic parasympathetic fibres. It is the competitive inhibitor of the muscarinic action of acetylcholine and is the strongest of drugs available for cycloplegic purposes.

Indications and Usage

- It is used for mydriasis and cycloplegia.
- Pupillary dilation in inflammatory conditions of the iris
- Amblyopia therapy.

Contraindications

Contraindicated in persons with primary glaucoma or a tendency towards glaucoma, e.g. narrow anterior chamber angle and in those persons showing hypersensitivity to any component of this preparation.

Precautions

To avoid excessive systemic absorption the lacrimal sac should be compressed for one minute after instillation.

Adverse Reactions

Local: Atropine can cause allergic responses, usually around the eyelids and conjunctiva. The allergic responses include redness and crusty flaking of the eyelid margins, dryness and wrinkling of the skin around the eyelids and injected bulbar conjunctiva with some watery discharge. Blurred vision and photophobia are consequent to the cycloplegic and mydriatic effect of phenylephrine.

Systemic: Dryness of skin and mouth, tachycardia, skin rash. Abdominal distension in infants and hyperpyrexia may occur in children. Severe reactions are manifested by hypotension with progressive respiratory depression. The elderly are more susceptible to anticholinergic toxicity like cognitive impairment, delirium and hallucinations.

Plasma concentrations peak after 10 min of topical application. Two drops of 1% solution contain 1 mg of the drug which is twice the preoperative injectable dose.

Dosage and Administration

Because of a long duration of its effect and delay in the onset of action it is not routinely used for office procedures.

In children—For refraction, administer one or two drops 0.5% solution to each eye, twice daily for one to three days prior to examination.

HOMATROPINE HYDROBROMIDE
(Homide)

Description

Homatropine 2% sterile ophthalmic solution was the first anticholinergic to be developed specifically as an alternative to atropine.

It is a synthetic anticholinergic agent that directly blocks the muscarinic action of acetylcholine, causing mydriasis and cycloplegia. Its effect generally lasts longer than those of either cyclopentolate or tropicamide but it is not necessarily more effective. Homatropine is therefore not commonly used as diagnostic agent, however, its relatively long-lasting effect makes it valuable in the treatment of anterior ocular inflammations such as iritis.

Indications and Usage

A moderately long-acting mydriatic and cycloplegic agent for cycloplegic refraction and in the treatment of inflammatory condition of the uveal tract. It is inferior to atropine for penalization therapy of amblyopia.

Contraindications

In persons with a tendency of occludable angles. It should not be used in patients who have shown allergy to atropine.

Warning

Patient should be advised not to drive or engage in other hazardous activities while pupils are dilated. Caution also in pregnant and lactating mothers.

Adverse Reactions

Adverse reactions are similar to atropine but much less in frequency. Prolonged use may produce local irritation characterized by follicular conjunctivitis, vascular congestion, edema, exudate and an eczematoid dermatitis.

Dosage and Administration

For refraction instill one or two drops topically in the eye(s). May be repeated in 5 to 10 minutes if necessary.

CYCLOPENTOLATE HYDROCHLORIDE
(Cyclogyl)

Description

Cyclopentolate 1% is an anticholinergic prepared as a sterile ophthalmic solution. Also available as 0.5% and 2% solution.

Indications

Cyclopentolate is an effective antimuscarinic agent and the cycloplegic of choice for children under age 12 when latent hyperopia or accommodative esotropia is suspected. Its cycloplegic efficacy is greater than homatropine. Also used for pre- and postoperative states when mydriasis is required and when a short-acting mydriatic cycloplegic is needed in the therapy of iridocyclitis. Unlike atropine and homatropine onset of maximum cycloplegia approximates the onset of maximum mydriasis.

Contraindications

Narrow angle glaucoma and in patients with hypersensitivity to the drug. Cyclopentolate is also not recommended for children with emotional problems since it can have marked central nervous system effects that may be increased in susceptible youngsters.

Dosage and Administration

One drop followed by second drop in 5 minutes or as desired by the physician. Complete recovery usually occurs in 24 hours.

Adverse Reactions

Local: Increased intraocular pressure, blurred vision, photophobia.

Systemic: Psychotic reactions, behavioral disturbances seizures, disorientation and cardio-respiratory collapse in children have been reported. Dryness of the mouth, tachycardia, headache or allergic reaction may occur. Because toxic reactions occur with multiple instillations of 1% solution, the smallest dose should be used.

Management of over dosage in life-threatening toxicity includes slow injection of physostigmine intravenously.

TROPICAMIDE
(Tmide, Tropicacyl)

Description

Tropicamide is one of the most commonly used anticholinergic mydriatic because of its powerful mydriatic effects, rapid action and low incidence of side effects. It is available as 0.5% or 1% eyedrops.

Tropicamide acts by blocking muscaranic acetylcholine receptors. The stronger preparation (1%) also paralyses accommodation. The 0.5% strength may be useful in producing mydriasis with only slight cycloplegia.

Indications and Usage

For mydriasis and cycloplegia, for diagnostic procedures and when a short-acting mydriatic is needed for some pre- and postoperative stages. Unlike atropine, homatropine and cyclopentolate, pupillary dilation with tropicamide is less dependant on iris pigmentation. For premature infants a combination of 2.5% phenylephrine and 0.5% tropicamide is recommended because the latter alone fails to dilate adequately.

Contraindications

Contraindicated in narrow angle glaucoma and in persons showing hypersensitivity to any component of this preparation.

Precautions

In the elderly and others where increased intraocular pressure may be encountered, mydriatics and cycloplegics should be used with caution. This preparation may cause CNS disturbances that may be dangerous in infants and children.

Patient should be advised not to drive or engage in other hazardous activities while pupils are dilated.

Dosage and Administration

One or two drops of 1% solution in each eye 2 to 3 times at 5 minutes intervals or as directed by the physician.

Adverse Reactions

Local: Stinging sensation on instillation is very common.

Systemic: Rarely in children confusion or hyperactivity may occur.

Onset and recovery of cycloplegics

Drug	Strength of solution%	Mydriasis		Paralysis of accommodation	
		Maximal	Recovery	Maximal	Recovery
Atropine	1%	30–40 min	7–10 days	1–3 hr	6–12 days
Homatropine	2%	30–40 min	1–3 days	30–60 min	1–3 days
Cyclopentolate	0.5–1%	30–60 min	24 hr	30–60 min	24 hr
Tropicamide	0.5–1.0%	20–40 min	6 hr	30 min	6 hr

7

Antiglaucoma Agents

PILOCARPINE NITRATE/HYDROCHLORIDE
(Pilocar)

Description

Pilocarpine nitrate, is a topical parasympathomimetic agent which duplicates the muscuranic effects of acetylcholine, but has no nicotinic effect. Available as 1%, 2% or 4% drops. Since the drug is bound to melanin higher doses are needed in pigmented eyes. Pilocarpine is effective in the treatment of glaucoma by improving the facility of outflow. It is very stable and has a long shelf life.

Indications and Usage

Indicated for:

- The control of intraocular pressure in glaucoma
- Emergency relief of mydriasis in an acutely glaucomatous situation
- To reverse mydriasis caused by a cycloplegic agent.

Contraindications

Pilocarpine is contraindicated in persons showing hypersensitivity to any of its components, in acute inflammatory conditions of the anterior segment, some forms of secondary glaucoma.

Precautions

Pilocarpine has been reported to cause retinal detachment in individuals with pre-existing retinal diseases or predisposed to retinal tears. Safety and effectiveness in children have not been established. Caution is also advised in patients of bronchial asthma, parkinsonism and peptic ulcer.

Adverse Reactions

Include visual blurring due to miosis and accommodative spasm, poor dark adaptation caused by the failure of the pupil to dilate in reduced illumination and conjunctival hyperemia. Headache and browache may occur due to ciliary spasm. Miotics have been reported to cause lens opacities in susceptible individuals after prolonged use.

Prolonged use of antiglaucoma drugs has been found to alter conjunctival tissue and increase the failure chances of trabeculectomy.

Dosage and Administration

For glaucoma: The recommended dosage is 1 to 2 drops two to four times a day of the selected concentration, patient response may be variable. Onset of IOP reduction occurs within an hour.

It is also available in gel form. A single 4% pilocarpine gel at bedtime is equivalent to using a 4% solution 4 times/day.

PHOSPHOLINE IODIDE

Description

Phospholine iodide occurs as a white crystalline water-soluble hygroscopic solid having a slight merceptar like odours. It is available in the following concentrations: 0.03%, 0.06%, 0.125%, 0.25%.

Actions

Phospholine iodide is a long-acting cholinesterase inhibitor for topical use which enhances the effect of endogenously liberated acetycholine of iris, ciliary muscle and other parasympathetically innervated structures of the eye. It thereby causes miosis, increase in facility of aqueous humor, fall in intraocular pressure and potentiation of accommodation.

Indications

In chronic open angle glaucoma, sub-acute or chronic angle closure glaucoma after iridotomy or where surgery is refused or contraindicated. When applied topically at the lid margins it can effectively remove the crab louse but not their nits.

Contraindications

- Active uveal inflammation.
- Most cases of angle closure glaucoma due to the possibility of increasing angle block.
- Hypersensitivity to the active or inactive ingredients.

Adverse Reactions

- Stinging, burning, lacrimation, lid muscle twitching conjunctival and ciliary redness, browache, induced myopia with visual blurring may occur.
- Activation of latent iritis or uveitis may occur.
- Iris cysts may form and if treatment is continued may enlarge and obscure vision. This occurrence is more frequent in children.
- Prolonged use may cause conjunctival thickening, obstruction of nasolacrimal canals.
- Lens opacities, paradoxical increase in intraocular pressure.

Dosage and Administration

Early chronic glaucoma, 0.03% instilled twice a day.

EPINEPHRINE BITARTARATE
(Epitrate)

Description

Epinephrine bitartrate ophthalmic solution is a sterile aqueous solution of levorotatory epinephrine bitartrate, available as 1% or 2% concentration.

Mechanism of Action

Epinephrine bitartrate lowers intraocular pressure by reducing the rate of aqueous formation. Improvement in outflow facility is also observed in certain cases following prolonged therapy.

Indications and Usage

Useful in the treatment of open angle glaucoma, especially in young persons who may be troubled by miotic induced accommodative spasms. It can also be used in older cataractous patients who may experience poor vision with a miotic pupil.

Contraindications

Contraindicated in persons with narrow angles. Also it should not be used in patients taking monoamine oxidase inhibitors or tricyclic antidepressants, since severe hypertensive reactions can result.

Warnings

Topical use of epinephrine in any form should be interrupted prior to general anesthesia with certain anesthetics such as cyclopropane or halothane, which sensitize the myocardium to sympathomimetics. It should be used in caution in hypertensives and hyperthyroid patients.

Adverse Reactions

Local: Transitory stinging on initial instillation may be expected because of low pH. Headache or browache frequently occurs on beginning this therapy but usually diminish as the treatment is continued. Pigmentary deposits in the lids, conjunctiva or cornea may occur after prolonged use. Epidermalization of the lacrimal punctum has been reported. It may induce a macular edema especially in aphakic and pseudophakic eyes.

Systemic: Elevation of blood pressure, tachycardia, arrhythmias, tremor, and headaches are consequences of the adrenergic effect.

Dosage and Administration

One drop with frequency of instillation being individualized from every two or three days to twice daily. More frequent instillation than one drop four times daily does not usually elicit any further improvement in therapeutic responses.

DIPIVEFRIN HYDROCHLORIDE
(Propine)

Description

It is a lipophilic prodrug derivative of epinephrine.

Mechanism of Action

It is similar to epinephrine.

Indications

For the control of intraocular pressure in chronic open angle glaucoma or ocular hypertensive patients with open angles. IOP reduction occurs to the extent of 20–30%. Dipivefrin has been used successfully in patients who have demonstrated intolerance to epinephrine.

Contraindications

The safety of the intensive or protracted use of dipivefrin during pregnancy has not been established. Contraindicated in patients suffering from closed angle glaucoma.

Macular edema is a rare occurrence with adrenaline use in aphakic patients. Prompt reversal generally follows the discontinuation of the drug.

Adverse Reactions

Local: Rebound vasodilatation and allergic blepharo-conjunctivitis are rarely observed following treatment with dipivefrin. Adrenochrome deposits have been rarely observed following the use of dipivefrin. Very slight transitory stinging may occur upon instillation in some patients. Dipivefrin does not cause macular edema in aphakic eyes as does epinephrine, but should be avoided as first line drug in these eyes.

Systemic: As concentration of dipivefrin is one-tenth that of epinephrine, cardiovascular side effects are less problematic.

Dosage

The usual dosage is one drop (0.1%) in the affected eye(s) every 12 hours. Peak effect occurs in 4 hours. Patient should be instructed to occlude the lacrimal punctum to avoid systemic absorption of the drug.

TIMOLOL
(Glucomol, Nyolol, Iotim)

Description

Timolol (Timolol Maleate) ophthalmic solution is a non-selective beta-adrenergic receptor blocking agent available as 0.25% and 0.5% concentration. Timolol maleate possesses an asymmetric carbon atom in its structure and is provided as the laevoisomer.

Timolol is stable at room temperature.

Clinical Pharmacology

Timolol maleate is a beta$_1$ and beta$_2$ (non-selective) adrenergic receptor blocking agent that does not have significant intrinsic sympathomimetic, or local anesthetic (membrane-stabilizing) activity.

Beta-adrenergic receptor blockade reduces cardiac output in both healthy subjects and patients with heart disease. In patients with severe impairment of myocardial function beta-adrenergic receptor blockade may inhibit the stimulatory effect of the sympathetic nervous system necessary to maintain adequate cardiac function. Beta-adrenergic receptor blockade in the bronchi and bronchioles results in increased airway resistance from unopposed para-sympathetic activity. Such an effect in patients with asthma or other bronchospastic conditions is potentially dangerous.

Timolol ophthalmic solution, when applied topically in the eye, has the action of reducing elevated as well as normal intraocular pressure, whether or not accompanied by glaucoma. The onset of reduction in intraocular pressure following administration of timolol can usually be detected within half an hour after a single dose. The maximum effect usually occurs in one to two hours and significant lowering of intraocular pressure can be maintained for periods as long as 24 hours with a single dose. Repeated observations over a period of one year indicate that the intraocular pressure-lowering effect of timolol is well maintained.

Tonography and fluorophotometry studies in man suggest that its predominant action may be related to reduced aqueous formation. However, in some studies a slight increase in outflow facility was also observed.

Indications and Usage

Timolol Ophthalmic Solution has been shown to be effective in lowering intraocular pressure in both primary and secondary glaucomas.

Clinical trials have shown that IOP reduction with timolol twice a day was 31–33% compared to 22% with pilocarpine 4% four times a day and 28% with epinephrine.

Contraindications

Timolol is contraindicated in patients with bronchial asthma or severe chronic obstructive pulmonary disease, sinus bradycardia; second and third degree atrioventricular block overt cardiac failure; cardiogenic shock; hypersensitivity to any component of this product.

Warnings

As with other topically applied ophthalmic drugs, this drug may be absorbed systemically. The same adverse reactions found with systemic administration of beta-adnergic blocking agents may occur with topical administration. Death due to bronchospasm in patients with asthma and rarely death in association with cardiac failure, have been reported following administration of timolol.

Timolol and other beta-adrenergic blocking agents should be administered with caution in patients subject to spontaneous hypoglycemic or to diabetic patients (especially those with labile diabetes who are receiving insulin or oral hypoglycema agents). Beta-adrenergic receptor blocking agents may mask the signs and symptoms of acute hypoglycemia.

Beta-adrenergic blocking agents may also mask certain clinical signs (e.g. tachycardia) of hyperthyroidism. Patients suspected of developing thyrotoxicosis should be managed carefully to avoid abrupt withdrawal of beta-adrenergic blocking agents which might precipitate a thyroid storm.

Muscle weakness: Beta-adrenergic blockade has been reported to potentiate muscle weakness consistent with certain myasthenic symptoms (e.g., diplopia, ptosis and generalized weakness).

As respiratory and cardiovascular side effects may also occur in infants and children timolol should be used with caution.

Drug Interactions

Patients who are receiving a beta-adrenergic blocking agent orally and timolol should be observed for a potential additive effect either on the intraocular pressure or on the known systemic effects of beta blockage.

Although timolol used alone has little or no effect on pupil size, mydriasis resulting from concomitant therapy with timolol and epinephrine has been reported occasionally. When used with an adrenergic agonist it might happen that timolol may antagonise the effect of the adrenergic agonist, hence it must be administered after 2–3 hours of administering the adrenergic agonist.

Close observation of the patient is recommended when a beta blocker is administered to patients receiving catecholamine- depleting drugs such as reserpine, because of possible additive effects and the production of hypotension and/or marked bradycardia, which may produce vertigo, syncope, or postural hypotension.

Co-administration of calcium antagonists and digitalis can induce atrioventricular conduction disturbances.

Adverse Reactions

Local: Ocular irritation, decreased corneal sensitivity.
Systemic: Cardiovascular Bradycardia, arrhythmia, hypotension, syncope, heart block, cerebral vascular accident, cerebral ischemia, congestive heart failure, palpitation. *Digestive* Nausea, *nervous system* headache, Dizziness *Psychiatric* Depression *Skin* Hypersensitivity, including localized and generalized rash urticaria.

Respiratory Bronchospasm (predominantly in patients with pre-existing chronic obstructive pulmonary disease), respiratory failure. *Others:* Include aggravation of myathenic symptoms, sexual dysfunction, masking of hypoglycemic symptoms in diabetics.

Over Dosage

No data are available with regard to over dosage in humans. An in vitro hemodialysis study, using timolol added to human plasma or whole body, showed that timolol was readily dialyzed from these fluids; however, a study of patients with renal failure showed that timolol did not dialyse readily.

The most common signs and symptoms to be expected with over-dosage with administration of a systemic beta-adrenergic receptor blocking agent is symptomatic bradycardia, hypotension, bronchospasm and acute cardiac failure. The following additional therapeutic measures should be considered:

- *Gastric lavage:* If ingested.
- *Symptomatic bradycardia:* Use atropine sulfate intravenously in a dosage of 0.25 mg to 2 mg to induce vagal blockade. If bradycardia persists, intravenous isoproterenol hydrochloride should be administered cautiously. In refractory cases the use of a transvenous cardiac pacemaker may be considered.
- *Hypotension:* Use sympathomimetic presser drug therapy, such as dopamine, dobutamine or levarterenol. In refractory cases the use of glucagon hydrochloride has been reported to be useful.
- *Bronchospasm:* Use isoproterenol hydrochloride. Additional therapy with aminophylline may be considered.
- *Acute cardiac failure:* Conventional therapy with digitalis, diuretics and oxygen should be instituted immediately. In refractory cases the use of intravenous aminophylline is suggested. This may be followed if necessary to be useful.
- *Heart block (second or third degree):* Use isoproterenol hydrochloride or a transvenous cardiac pacemaker.

Dosage and Administration

Timolol ophthalmic solution is available in concentrations of 0.25 and 0.5 percent. The usual starting dose is one drop of 0.25 percent timolol in the affected eye (s) twice a day. If the clinical response is not adequate, the dosage may be changed to one drop of 0.5 percent solution in the affected eye (s) twice a day. Since in some patients the pressure-lowering response to timolol may require a few weeks to stabilize, evaluation should include a determination of intraocular pressure after approximately 4 weeks of treatment with timolol.

CARTEOLOL HYDROCHLORIDE
(Ocupress)

Description

Carteolol hydrochloride is a non-cardio-selective. Topical beta-blocker with the advantage of intrinsic sympathomimetic activity. Available as sterile eyedrops containing carteolol hydrochloride 1% or 2% w/v. Compared to timolol which is lipophilic, carteolol is hydrophilic requiring greater concentration for corneal penetration.

Contraindications

Uncontrolled cardiac insufficiency, bronchospasm, bronchial asthma, chronic obstructive pulmonary disease, pregnancy, hypersensitivity.

Precautions

As with other topically applied ophthalmic preparations, carteolol may be absorbed systemically. Therefore, it should be used with caution in patients receiving systemic beta-blockers or with known contraindications to systemic beta blocker, e.g. sinus bradycardia, second and third degree block, cardiogenic shock, uncontrolled diabetes. Carteolol Hydrochloride may be systemically absorbed and penetrate the breast milk. Use in lactating mothers should therefore be at the discretion of the physician.

Side Effects

Local: Ocular reactions such as irritation, burning, pain blurred vision, conjunctival hyperemia and corneal disorders such as keratitis may occasionally develop.

Systemic: Adverse events are similar to those reported with timolol. As with all beta-blockers, bradycardia, dyspnoea, headache, asthenia and vertigo have occasionally been reported.

Dosage and Administration

Initially the recommended adult dose is one drop of carteolol 1% eyedrops in affected eye twice daily. If required the dosage may be altered to one drop of carteolol 2% eyedrops in affected eyes twice daily.

LEVOBUNOLOL
(Betagan)

Description

It is a non-cardio selective beta-blocker. Levobunolol is 60 times more potent than its dextro isomer.

Indications

Where IOP reduction is desired, its efficacy is similar to that of timolol.

Contraindications

Same as for timolol.

Warnings

Same as for timolol. The solution should be used within one month of opening the container.

Adverse Reactions

Same as for timolol. Incidence of burning and stinging sensation with levobunolol is more as well as the incidence of blepharo-conjunctivitis compared to timolol. Compared to other topical beta blockers corneal anesthesia is not a significant problem.

There may be a decrease in resting heart rate by 3–10 heart beats/minute. There may be a mild decrease in blood pressure also.

Dosage and Administration

One drop once or twice daily. The onset of action can be detected within an hour after treatment with maximum effect seen between 2 and 6 hours. A significant IOP lowering can be maintained for up to 24 hours after a single dose.

BETAXOLOL HYDROCHLORIDE
(Optipres, Iobet)

Description

Betaxolol hydrochloride is the only (β_1) cardioselective ophthalmic beta-blocker.

Indications

IOP reduction in primary and secondary glaucomas and ocular hypertension. IOP reduction is about 25% from baseline values which is marginally lower compared to timolol.

Contraindications

Betaxolol is contraindicated in patients with sinus bradycardia greater than a first degree block, cardiogenic shock or a history of cardiac failure and in patients with hypersensitivity to any component.

Warnings

Patients who are receiving beta-adrenergic blocking agents orally and betaxolol should be observed for potential additive effect either on intraocular pressure or the known systemic effects of beta blockade. While betaxolol, has demonstrated a low potential for systemic effects, it should be used with caution in patients with excessive restriction of pulmonary function, in patients with diabetes (especially labile diabetes) or in patients suspected of developing thyrotoxicosis. Consideration should be given to the gradual withdrawal of beta-adrenergic blocking agents prior to general anesthesia because of the reduced ability of the heart to respond to beta adrenergically mediated sympathetic reflex stimuli.

Adverse Reactions

Local: Although betaxolol is well tolerated, some patients upon instillation may experience discomfort of short duration and occasional tearing has been reported. Rare instances of decreased corneal sensitivity, itching, corneal punctate staining, keratitis, anisocoria and photophobia have been reported.

Systemic: Systemic reactions following topical administration of betaxolol (e.g. insomnia and depressive neurosis) have only rarely been reported.

Dosage and Administration

The usual dose (0.5%) is one drop instilled twice daily. The lower incidence of pulmonary side effects makes it a better choice for use in children, though no specific studies are available. However, the beta 1 adrenergic selectivity of betaxolol is only relative and the drug is capable of inducing pulmonary side effects in susceptible patients.

DORZOLAMIDE
(Trusopt)

Description

Dorzolamide hydrochloride is a carbonic anhydrase inhibitor available as 2% ophthalmic solution.

Like the oral agents it has a sulfonamide group that is essential for its activity and another amine group that gives it lipid-water solubility essential for corneal penetration.

Indications

It is used as monotherapy or in combination with other antiglaucoma agents specially beta blockers. Maximum IOP lowering is approximately 22%.

Contraindication

Hypersensitivity to any component of this preparation.

Adverse Effects

Ocular burning, stinging sensation and ocular irritation. Ocular allergy and superficial punctuate keratitis is seen in 10% patients.

Bitter taste has been reported with this drug in 25% patients.

Dosage

2% dorzolamide is instilled one drop in the affected eye three times a day. If another topical antiglaucoma agent is being used, administer the two at least ten minutes apart. It has been tried in children with no long-term adverse effects.

BRINZOLAMIDE
(Azopt)

Description

Available as 1% solution.

Mechanism of Action

Inhibition of carbonic anhydrase (CA) in the ciliary processes of the eye reduces aqueous production. It is a highly selective CA II inhibitor.

Adverse Effects

Local: It causes less ocular irritation compared to dorzolamide.

Systemic: Though sulfonamide related side effects have not been reported with brinzolamide, they may occur. Bitter and unusual taste is reported in 5–10% patients.

Precautions

It is not recommended in patients receiving oral carbonic anhydrase inhibitors.

Dosage

One drop three times/day.

BRIMONIDINE
(Alphagan, Iobrim)

Description

It is an alpha adrenergic agonist with selectivity to alpha$_2$ receptors. It is available as brimonidine tartrate 0.2% solution with benzalkonium chloride preservative 0.05 mg. Recently it has been marketed as 0.15% and 0.1% solution. Purite is another preservative that has been used with the newer preprations. It is highly lipophilic with good corneal penetration.

Mechanism of Action

It inhibits aqueous humor formation and enhances uveoscleral outflow. It is known to have a contralateral effect on the other eye possibly through the CNS.

Indications

For chronic use in glaucoma. It can be used specifically for controlling IOP spikes occurring post YAG iridotomy, laser trabeculoplasty or post YAG capsulotomy. The IOP lowering is 20–30%.When added to timolol it has an additive effect.

Contraindications

It is contraindicated in patients on MAO inhibitor therapy and those who show hypersensitivity to the drug. It is not preferred in infants and very young children due to apnea and seizures reported.

Adverse Effects

Local: Incidence of allergic follicular conjunctivitis has been reported to occur in 10% to as high as 40% patients. Conjunctival blanching and later hyperemia occurs after instillation.

Systemic: Fatigue, drowsiness, dry mouth. Sleepiness and lethargy are relatively common side effects that the patient should be warned of.

Precautions

Should be used with caution in patients with depression, thrombangitis obliterans, and those with orthostatic hypotension. Since it contains benzalkonium chloride it should be used with caution in patients wearing soft contact lenses.

Dosage

One drop administered twice daily.

LATANOPROST
(Xalatan, Latoprost)

Description

Latanoprost is available as 0.005% topical ophthalmic solution.

Mechanism of Action

Latanoprost is a selective FP receptor agonist. It increases uveoscleral outflow around the obstructed trabecular pathway the aqueous humor percolates through the ciliary muscle, suprachoroidal space and the sclera instead of exiting the eye through the trabecular meshwork and Schlemm's canal.

Indications

Latanoprost is indicated for reduction of elevated IOP in patients with open angle glaucoma and ocular hypertension and chronic angle closure glaucoma who are intolerant to or have insufficiently responded other antiglaucoma drugs. Latanoprost has been found to produce a greater IOP reduction in patients with higher pretreatment IOP.

IOP reduction in the range of 30–37% has been reported.

Contraindications

Hypersensitivity to any component of this preparation.

Adverse Effects

Local: Burning and stinging sensation, conjunctival hyperemia and punctate epithelial keratopathy, increased iris pigmentation increased eyelash growth. May induce cystoid macular edema in aphakics and those with uveitis. Hence it is not preferred in inflammatory glaucomas.

Systemic: Upper respiratory tract infection, migraine headache.

Dosage

Usual dosage is to instill one drop in the affected eyes once daily preferably in the evening. Reduction of IOP begins to occur 3–4 hours after administration and maximum effect is reached after 8–12 hours. The response lasts for 24 hours.

Precautions

Latanoprost ophthalmic solution is to be stored in refrigerator at 2–8°C when unopened. Once opened it may be stored at room temperature up to 25°C for 6 weeks. When using topical preparations containing thiomersal avoid instilling latanoprost for 10–15 minutes otherwise precipitation may occur.

TRAVOPROST
(Travatan)

Description

It is a prostaglandin agonist that selectively acts on FP receptors. It is absorbed in the cornea as a prodrug and hydrolysed to its biologically active free acid. Available as 0.004% solution with 0.015% benzalkonium chloride preservative.

Mechanism of Action

Same as latanoprost.

Indications

Same as latanoprost.

Contraindications

Patients who are aphakic, pseudophakic or with iritis have been reported to develop macular edema and hence are relative contraindications to the use of prostaglandins.

Adverse Effects

Local: Ocular hyperemia is the most common. Others include eye discomfort, increased iris pigmentation.

Systemic: Upper respiratory tract infections, bronchitis and chest pain are rare systemic side effects.

Precautions

Store between 2–25°C and discard the container after 6 weeks of opening it.

Dosage

One drop in the evening.

UNOPROSTONE ISOPROPYL
(Rescula)

Description

It a prostaglandin $F_{2\alpha}$ analog that increases outflow of aqueous. It is available as 0.15% solution.

Mechanism of Action

Same as latanoprost.

Indications

Same as latanoprost.

Adverse Effects

Local: The most common adverse effect is stinging sensation, increased eyelash growth, and hyper-pigmentation of the skin around the eyes. May cause increased brown pigmentation of the iris. The change in iris color occurs slowly and may not be noticeable for months or years.

Systemic: Flu like syndrome.

Dosage

It is recommended to be given as 1 drop twice daily.

BIMATOPROST
(Lumigan, Careprost)

Description

It is a synthetic prostamide that mimics the naturally occurring prostamides. It is available as 0.03% ophthalmic solution. It can be stored in room temperature (15–25°C).

Mechanism of Action

Same as latanoprost.

Indications

It can reduce IOP from 33–40% from baseline in ocular hypertension, POAG, and chronic angle closure glaucoma. It has been used in patients not responding to latanoprost.

Adverse Effects

Local: Conjunctival hyperemia, eyelash growth, periocular pigmentation of the skin are the most common.

Systemic: Migraine headaches, flu like syndrome have been reported.

Dosage

One drop once in the evening.

TAFLUPROST
(Saflutan)

Description

It is a topical ophthalmic medication for glaucoma marketed as 0.0015% solution containing 15 μg tafluprost per ml. Both preservative free and preservative-containing preparations are marketed.

Pharmacology

It is a novel PGF2α derivative in which the 15-position hydroxyl group is substituted by 2 fluorine atoms. This structural change makes the molecule resistant to one of the pathways of metabolism (ketonization) and prolongs its duration of action. It has highly selective affinity for the FP receptor. It acts by increasing the uveoscleral outflow of aqueous humor. Has been shown to increase retinal arterial blood flow around the optic disc, as well as an increase in the blood flow in retinal tissue. Claimed to have less likelihood of iris and/or eyelid pigmentation.

Adverse Reactions

Conjunctival hyperemia, eyelash abnormalities, itching sensation, ocular irritation, and iris pigmentation have been associated with tafluprost.

Precautions

Caution should be exercised when used for aphakic eyes or in bronchial asthma patients.

Indications and Usage

It is indicated for open angle glaucoma and normal tension glaucoma.

Dosage and Administration

One drop is to be instilled in eye(s) once in the evening.

Combination Choices available for Glaucoma

(Used when response to a single drug is insufficient)

Brimonidine and Timolol

Brimodin-P, Brimolol, Combigan: Available in 5 ml vial; one drop to be instilled thrice daily in affected eye(s).

Dorzolamide and Timolol

Dorzox-T, Ocudor-T: Available in 5 ml vial; one drop to be instilled twice daily in affected eye(s).

Latanoprost and Timolol

Laprost plus, Xalacom, Latocom eye: Available in 2.5/3 ml vial; one drop to be instilled once daily in affected eye(s).

Bimatoprost and Timolol

Ganfort: Available in 5 ml vial; one drop to be instilled once daily in affected eye(s).

Travoprost and Timolol

Travocom: Available in 5 ml vial; one drop to be instilled once daily in affected eye(s).

SYSTEMIC ANTIGLAUCOMA DRUGS

GLYCEROL

Description

Glycerin 50% and 75% is an oral osmotic agent for reducing intraocular pressure. Hyperosmotic agents transfer fluid from the eye to the circulation thereby decreasing IOP.

Indications and Usage

Glycerin 50% or 75% is indicated in the treatment of glaucoma to interrupt acute attacks and when a temporary drop in pressure is required which cannot be readily obtained by other means.

Contraindications

Patients with anuria, frank pulmonary edema, or those with severe cardiac decompensation. Diabetes is a relative contraindication for the use of glycerol.

Precaution

Caution should be exercised in hypovolemia, confused mental states, congestive heart failure and in dehydrated patients such as the diabetic. Safety and effectiveness in children have not been established. Caution should be exercised while administering it before ocular surgery as it may induce nausea and vomiting. Administer cautiously in the elderly senile patients especially if there is a history of urinary retention and diabetic patients or those with a cardiac problem and in severely dehydrated individuals.

Adverse Reactions

Nausea, vomiting, headache, confusion and disorientation may occur. Severe dehydration, cardiac arrhythmia or hyperosmolar non-ketotic coma which may result in death have been reported.

Dosage and Administration

Administer 1–1.5 gm of glycerin/kg body weight orally (2–3 ml of 50% glycerol/kg body wt in three divided doses). Peak effect occurs on 1 to 1.5 hours after administration and lasts 5 hours.

Needs to be administered in a flavored vehicle like lemon juice to avoid the severe nausea.

ISOSORBIDE

Description

Isosorbide 45% w/v oral solution is a dihydric alcohol prepared in a flavoured vehicle.

Isosorbide is readily absorbed after oral administration. It is essentially non-metabolized, and in the circulation, until it is eliminated by the kidney unchanged. The physical action of isosorbide is similar to that of other osmotic agents.

Indications and Usage

For the short-term reduction of intraocular pressure to interrupt an acute attack of glaucoma. May be used prior to and after intraocular surgery. Use where less risk of nausea and vomiting than that posed by other oral hyperosmotic agents is needed.

Contraindications

Same as for glycerol. However, it is relatively safer in diabetics than glycerol.

Warnings

With repeated doses, consideration should be given to maintenance of adequate fluid and electrolyte balance.

If urinary output continues to decrease, the patient's clinical status should be closely reviewed. Accumulation of isosorbide may result in over expansion of the extra-cellular fluid.

Repetitive doses should be used with caution particularly in patients with diseases associated with salt retention. Ensure that patients bladder has been emptied prior to surgery.

Adverse Reactions

Nausea, vomiting, headache, confusion and disorientation may occur. Very rare occurrences of syncope, gastric discomfort, lethargy, vertigo, thirst, dizziness, hiccups, hyperosmolarity, irritability, rash and light headedness have been reported.

Dosage and Administration

The recommended initial dose 1.5 gm/kg body weight of isosorbide (45%). The onset of action is usually within 30 min. while the maximum effect is expected at 1 to 1½ hours and lasts 3–5 hours.

MANNITOL

Description

It is currently the most commonly used intravenous hyperosmotic agent. Mannitol is more useful than urea as an intravenously administered osmotic agent for reducing intraocular pressure.

Mechanism of Action

The mannitol molecule is three times larger than that of urea, but it exerts a comparable osmotic effect, since mannitol is concentrated in the extracellular fluid compartments, which contain only one-third of the total body water. As with urea, the mannitol induced pressure lowering effect coincides with the increase in serum osmotic pressure. This ocular hypotensive effect occurs in 30–60 min depending on the rate of infusion, and lasts for about 6 hours. Because of vitreous dehydration, the anterior chamber deepens with intravenous infusion of mannitol as with urea.

Contraindications

Patients in renal failure or with congestive heart failure.

Precautions

Patients with impaired cardiovascular status may suddenly decompensate with a congestive heart failure. By a diuresis, mannitol may intensify inadequate hydration or hypo-volemia. Sodium potassium measurements are therefore important in monitoring patients on combination of oral acetazolamide, glycerol and mannitol. Intense diuresis after mannitol may lead to urinary retention and a need for catheterization especially in men with prostatic hyperplasia.

Adverse Effects

All osmotic agents may produce headache, dizziness and backache, presumably from cerebral dehydration and decreased cerebrospinal fluid volume. Dryness of mouth and increased thirst often occur. Fluid and electrolyte imbalance (hypokalemia) and acidosis may occur.

Dosage and Administration

Mannitol solutions tend to crystallize at cooler temperatures. The crystals will go back into solution if the containers is warmed, hence shake the bottle well before using. Do not freeze. To avoid crystals one can use the blood administration filter in the infusion line.

Mannitol dosage is 2 g/kg of a 20% solution given intravenously during a 30 minute period (7–10 ml/kg). The rate of administration may vary from 20 to 45 minutes. Peak IOP reduction occurs 1–1.5 hours after administration. The duration of IOP reduction is 2–6 hours.

ACETAZOLAMIDE
(Diamox, Iopar SR)

Description

Acetazolamide is a carbonic anhydrase inhibitor that is effective in slowing the production of aqueous humor by as much as sixty percent. Available as 125 and 250 mg tablets and 500 mg/vial.

Acetazolamide acts specifically on carbonic anhydrase, the enzyme which catalyzes the reversible reaction involving the hydration of carbon dioxide and the dehydration of carbonic acid. In the eye, this inhibitory action of acetazolamide decreases the secretion of aqueous humor and results in a drop in intraocular pressure, a reaction considered desired in cases of glaucoma and even in certain non-glaucomatous conditions. Based on reports that metabolic acidosis states reduce IOP, it is hypothesized that acetazolamide may act by inducing metabolic acidosis rather than directly through carbonic anhydrase inhibition.

The diuretic effect of acetazolamide is due to its action in the kidney involving hydration of carbonic dioxide and dehydration of carbonic acid. The result is renal loss of HCO_3 ion, which carries out sodium, water and potassium, alkalinization of the urine and promotion of diuresis are thus effected. However, urinary excretion of citrate is reduced which may lead to renal stones later.

Indications

In chronic simple (open angle) glaucoma, secondary glaucoma and preoperatively in acute angle closure glaucoma where delay of surgery is desired in order to lower intraocular pressure.

Contraindications

Acetazolamide therapy is contraindicated in situations in which sodium and potassium blood serum levels are depressed in cases of marked kidney and liver diseases or dysfunction.

Adverse Reactions

Adverse reactions during short-term therapy are minimal. Those effects which have been noted include paresthesias, particularly a tingling feeling in the extremities, some loss of appetite, taste alteration, transient myopia, polyuria, loss of libido and occasional instances of drowsiness and confusion. Other side effects include urticaria, hematuria, glycosuria, hepatic insufficiency, flaccid paralysis and convulsions.

Metabolic acidosis induced in children may cause feeding problems. Elderly patients are less tolerant to the adverse effects of acetazolamide, hence in them the initial dose should be low.

Warnings

Studies of acetazolamide in rats and mice have demonstrated teratogenic and embryocidal effects at doses in excess of ten times those recommended in human beings. There is no evidence of this effect in human beings. However, acetazolamide, should not be used in pregnancy.

Use with caution in patients on concomitant systemic steroids as hypokalemia may develop. Potassium supplements in the form of Pot Klor can be given 0.30 ml of Pot Klor is dissolved in a glass of water and should be given with meals. Concomitant use with salicyclates may result in accumulation and toxicity of carbonic anhydrase inhibitors leading to metabolic acidosis and CNS depression.

Patients having sulfonamide allergy should avoid carbonic anhydrase inhibitors. Patients of sickle cell anemia should avoid acetazolamide as the metabolic acidosis induced leads to hemoconcentration with further sickling.

Dosage and Administration

The preferred dosage is 250 mg every 4 hours. Peak effect occurs in 1–4 hours.

Sustained release oral preparations are available for administering 500 mg twice daily. Their peak effect occurs in 3–6 hours. For long-term therapy sustained release preparations are better tolerated.

Intravenous therapy may be used for rapid decrease of IOP within minutes. It should never be given intramuscularly due to pain caused.

Children: Oral: 5–10 mg/kg/day in divided doses. For children the tablets can be crushed and dissolved in hot water, avoid using glycerin or alcohol based vehicles.

Parenteral: 5–10 mg/kg/dose.

METHAZOLAMIDE

Description

Methazolamide is a white, crystalline powder, weak acid, slightly soluble in water. It is available as 50 mg tablets.

Methazolamide is a potent inhibitor of the enzyme carbonic anhydrase. It is absorbed somewhat slowly from the gastrointestinal tract and disappears more slowly from the plasma than does acetazolamide. Methazolamide does have a diuretic effect resulting in increase in urinary volume with the excretion of sodium potassium and chloride but it is less active than acetazolamide.

Indications

For adjunctive treatment of chronic simple (open angle) glaucoma, secondary glaucoma and preoperatively in acute angle closure glaucoma where delay of surgery is desired in order to lower, intraocular pressure.

Adverse Reactions

Anorexia, nausea, vomiting, malaise, fatigue, drowsiness, headache, vertigo, mental confusion, depression, etc. Most adverse reactions of methazolamide have been relatively mild in character and disappear upon withdrawal of the drug on adjustment of dosage.

Dosage and Administration

The effective therapeutic dose administrated in tablet form varies from 50 mg to 100 mg 2–3 times daily. The drug may be used concomitantly with miotic and osmotic agents. It is not available for parenteral use.

ANTIGLAUCOMA DRUGS IN PREGNANCY

The use of antiglaucoma drugs during pregnancy may present some potential risk to the developing baby. The challenge of treating glaucoma in pregnancy is luckily not faced very frequently as the incidence of glaucoma in child bearing age is relatively less. Nevertheless such presentations are faced in practice and cautious approach has to be taken.

β-adrenergic tone is important for maintenance of the heart rate in fetus. So β-blockers have the potential of being harmful, when used in pregnancy. Though the association has not been strongly established, there are some reports showing weak association of topical timolol use and foetal cardiac arrhythmia and apnea. The topical drug has the risk to produce some adverse effect after getting absorbed through the nasopharyngeal mucosa. So β-blockers should be avoided during pregnancy, especially in the first trimester.

Despite the experiments suggesting harmful effects in animals, among the miotics, pilocarpine has not been associated with birth defects in humans when used in early pregnancy. When used later in pregnancy it may cause weakness, fits and increased temperature in the newborn. Carbachol and ecothiophate have shown harmful effects in animals and may cause muscle weakness in the new born.

Early use of adrenaline can produce defects as cataract and hernia. Even the prodrug dipivefrine has to be used very cautiously. Apraclonidine has not shown any problem in preclinical animal studies but enough safety studies in humans is lacking. Brimonidine can cross the placenta. It has been associated with lowering of blood pressure and abortions.

Acetazolamide can also cross placenta to produce adverse effects such as metabolic acidosis, neonatal renal tubular acidosis, and neonatal teratoma. If necessary the blood levels of the drug should be monitored to prevent the overdose and the adverse effects. Enough studies about dorzolamide in pregnancy are lacking.

There are also controversial and conflicting opinions about use of prostaglandin analogues. While it is reported that latanoprost and travoprost do not have sufficient active harmful ingredients for the developing fetus and can be used safely other reports are inconclusive for their safety in pregnancy. Prostaglandins in general should be avoided in pregnancy because they can induce labor. In animal experiments these have found to be safe. Latanoprost even at high experimental doses has not been seen to cause adverse effects in growing fetus in animals.

So during pregnancy minimum necessary antiglaucoma drugs should be used in lowest possible concentrations and for minimum number of times per day. Systemic absorption of the drug can be reduced to much extent (by about two thirds of the instilled drug) by punctal occlusion. Alternatives to drugs like laser surgery should be considered.

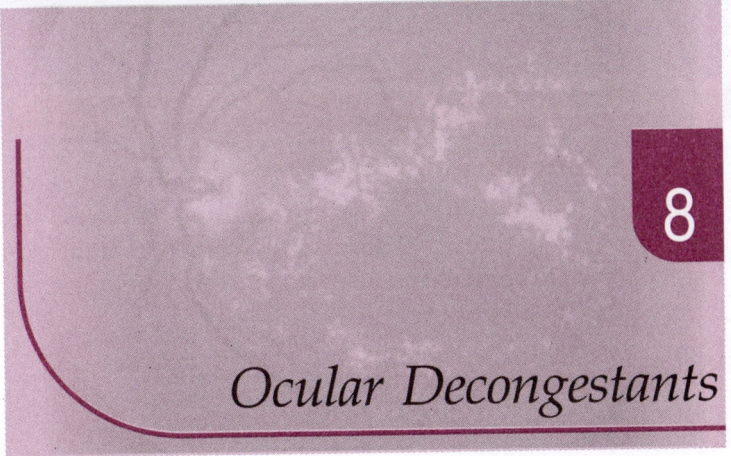

8

Ocular Decongestants

NAPHAZOLINE HYDROCHLORIDE
(Clearine, Mezol)

Description

An ocular vasoconstrictor prepared as 0.1% sterile topical ophthalmic solution.

Actions

Constricts the vasculature of the conjunctiva. It is presumed this effect is due to the direct action of the drug upon the alpha (excitatory) receptors of the vascular smooth muscles.

Indications

A topical ocular vasoconstrictor.

Contraindications

Hypersensitivity to a component of this medication.

Precautions

Use only with caution in the presence of hypertension, cardiac irregularities, hyperglycemia (diabetes) and hyperthyroidism. A severe hypertensive crisis may ensue in patients under MAO inhibitor medication from use of a sympathomimetic drug.

Adverse Reactions

Pupillary dilation with increase in intraocular pressure, systemic effects due to absorption. Accidental ingestion especially in children may cause marked sedation requiring emergency treatment.

Dosage and Administration

1–2 drops every 3–4 hours.

TETRAHYDROZOLINE HYDROCHLORIDE
(Visine)

Description

Terahydrozoline hydrochloride is a sterile, isotonic buffered ophthalmic solution containing 0.05% tetrahydrozoline hydrochloride.

Indications

Tetrahydrozoline is a decongestant ophthalmic solution designed to provide symptomatic relief of conjunctival edema and hyperemia secondary to ocular allergics, minor irritations and so-called nonspecific or catarrhal conjunctivitis. Beneficial effects include amelioration of burning, irritation, pruritus, soreness and excessive lacrimation.

Contraindications

Hypersensitivity to one or more component of this preparation.

Adverse Reactions

The following adverse reactions may be observed pupillary dilation, increase in intraocular pressure, systemic effects due to absorption (i.e. hypertension cardiac irregularities, hyperglycemia, etc.) may occur at very high doses.

Dosage and Administration

1–2 drops instilled in each eye 3–4 times daily.

9

Immunosuppressive/ Antineoplastic Agents

Common Immunosuppressive/ Antineoplastic Agents

Antimetabolites	Azathioprine
	Methotrexate
	5-fluorouracilmercaptopurine
Alkylating agents	Cyclophosphamide
	Chlorambucil
	Mechlorthamine
	Triethylene thiophosphoramide
Antibiotic immuno-suppresants	Cyclosporine
Immunomodulating antibodies	Infliximab
	Imiquimod
Mitotic inhibitors	Vincristine
	Etoposide

AZATHIOPRINE
(Imuran)

Description

Azathioprine is a derivative of 6-mercaptopurine in which substitution of the sulfhydryl group has been achieved to impede degradation of the compound in vivo.

Actions

Azathioprine is an antimetabolite that acts by interfering with nucleic acid synthesis. It has been used in the treatment of thrombocytopenic purpura, autoimmune hemolytic anemia, glomerulonephritis, lupus erythematous, polymyositis, Crohn's disease, and rheumatoid arthritis. Antibody formation is inhibited by azathioprine, for this reason, the drug has been used in suppressing immune reactions after whole organ transplantation.

Ophthalmic Uses

Azathioprine has been used experimentally and in a limited number of clinical cases to suppress immune reactions in the cornea and uvea.

Adverse Effects

Azathioprine may produce nausea, vomiting, leukopenia and bone marrow depression. Increased susceptibility to many common infections develops.

Dosage

Azathioprine tablet is available in 50 mg tablets. Azathioprine sodium is available as a 100 mg powder (lyophilized) for intravenous use.

1 to 1.5 mg/kg orally per day is given. Up to 150 mg can be given per day depending on the condition.

MERCAPTOPURINE
(Purinethol)

Description

Mercaptopurine is an analogue and metabolic antagonist of adenine, a nucleic acid constituent.

Actions

Mercaptopurine interferes with nucleic acid synthesis. It is also used in the treatment of acute leukemia and chronic mylocytic leukemia. Mercaptopurine suppresses antibody synthesis and has been used in the treatment of serious immune reactions.

Ophthalmic Uses

Mercaptopurine has been used to treat severe cases of uveitis unresponsive to corticosteroid and ACTH therapy.

Adverse Effects

Mercaptopurine is a cytotoxic agent and can produce many serious side reactions, including bone marrow depression, liver damage with jaundice, gastrointestinal irritation and ulceration, nausea, vomiting and anorexia. This drug can produce abortion and teratogenic effects, whenever possible, it should be avoided during the first trimester of pregnancy.

Dosage

It is available in the form of 50 mg tablets. The dosage is 2.5 to 5 mg/kg of body weight/day. Low doses should be used initially and increased if no clinical improvement occurs. Larger doses are used in the treatment of non-hematological malignancies.

METHOTREXATE
(Neotrexate)

Description

Methotrexate is a competitive inhibitor of the enzyme folic acid reductase, which reduces folic acid to tetrahydrofolic acid. It is a cytotoxic antifolate.

Mechanism of Action

Inhibits the enzyme dihydrofolate reductase, which is important in maintaining the levels of tetrahydrofolate cofactors necessary for one carbon transfer reactions in the synthesis of purines and thymidylate.

Its immunosuppressant action is due to inhibition of T-cell and B-cell proliferation.

Tetrahydrofolic acid is very important in DNA synthesis and cellular replication. Methotrexate inhibits the formation of tetrahydrofolic acid. Methotrexate is effective in the treatment of leukemias, Burkitt's tumor and various carcinomas. It is also used in the treatment of severe psoriasis.

Ophthalmic Uses

Methotrexate has been used in the treatment of severe forms of uveitis, including sympathetic ophthalmia.

Adverse Effects

Methotrexate may produce serious side effects including stomatitis, hemorrhagic enteritis, bone marrow suppression and hepatic dysfunction.

Dosage

Methotrexate is prepared in tablets 2.5 mg, powder 20 mg, solution 2 and 2.5 mg/ml.

Orally—2.5 to 5 mg/kg of body weight daily for 4 to 5 days, or twice weekly.

MECHLORETHAMINE
(Mustine HCL)

Actions

Mechlorethamine hydrochloride is a cytotoxin that has an affinity for cancer cells and other rapidly growing cells. The precise action of the drug is unknown. However, it interferes with growth and mitotic cell division. It is also used as a palliative agent in patients with Hodgkin's disease, lymphosarcoma, reticular cell sarcoma, and bronchogenic carcinoma.

Ophthalmic Uses

Mechlorethamine hydrochloride has been used in combination with X-ray therapy for the treatment of retinoblastoma. However, it has not been used as extensively in the treatment of this disorder as has triethylene melamine (TEM).

Adverse Effects

Nausea, vomiting, anorexia and thrombophlebitis are the common side effects. Others include lymphocytopenia, granulocytopenia, thrombocytopenia and anemia. Extravasation outside the vein leads to severe local inflammation and sometimes to sloughing of the overlying tissues.

Dosage

The preparation for injection is powder 10 mg.

The dosage is 0.1 to 0.3 mg/kg of body weight by intravenous injection daily for 4 days.

CHLORAMBUCIL
(Leukeran)

Description and Actions

Chlorambucil is a derivative of nitrogen mustard. It is cytotoxic and has been used in the treatment of chronic lymphotic leukemia, lymphomas, lymphosarcomas, and Hodgkin's disease. It is thought to be less toxic to the hemopoietic system than nitrogen mustard.

Ophthalmic Uses

Chlorambucil has been used in the treatment of severe immune inflammatory disorders such as uveitis and retinal vasculitis that have been unresponsive to corticosteroid therapy.

Adverse Effects

Bone marrow depression, including leukopenia, thrombocytopenia and anemia often occurs. This toxicity appears to be dose related and is usually reversible. Patients receiving chlorambucil should be monitored with regular blood counts. The drug is teratogenic and should not be used during the first trimester of pregnancy.

Preparation and Dosage

Chlorambucil 2 mg tablets should be given orally, usually adult dosage is 0.1 to 0.2 mg/kg of body weight for 3 to 6 weeks. Further treatment is defined by the response of patient and toxic reactions.

CYCLOPHOSPHAMIDE
(Endoxan)

Description

Cyclophosphamide is an antineoplastic drug related to nitrogen mustards. It is classified as an alkylating agent.

Actions

The exact mechanism of action of cyclophosphamide is unknown, it is probable the drug acts by interfering with DNA replication and cell division. It is useful in the treatment of Hodgkin's disease, lymphosarcoma, reticulum cell sarcoma, multiple myeloma and some forms of leukemia. The drug has also been used to suppress severe immune reactions including those after whole organ transplantation and severe disabling rheumatoid arthritis.

Ophthalmic Uses

Cyclophosphamide has been used to suppress severe uveitis especially posterior uveitis. It has also been used in the treatment of retinoblastoma.

Adverse Effects

Alopecia is a common side reaction, this is reversible. Leukopenia and bone marrow depression generally occurs. Other side reactions include nausea, vomiting, anorexia, weight loss, diarrhoea and mucosal ulceration. The drug is highly teratogenic.

Preparations and Dosage

Preparations include the following: Vials of 100 mg and 200 mg for injection and tablet 25 mg and 50 mg.

For antiinflammatory therapy, 50 mg is given daily and increased by 50 mg every four weeks until there is clinical improvement. The maintenance dose is 50 to 100 mg daily. A blood count should be obtained weekly and the leukocyte count maintained between 2500 and 5000/mm³.

TRIETHYLENE THIOPHOSPHORAMIDE (THIOTEPA)

Description

Triethylene thiophosphoramide is an alkylating agent related to nitrogen mustard.

Actions

The drug is used as a palliative agent in the treatment of neoplastic disease. Its action is believed to result from the release of ethylenimine radicals and their effects on dividing cells. The drug may be injected into local sites or given intravenously for the treatment of neoplasms.

Ophthalmic Uses

Triethylene thiophosphoramide has been applied topically to prevent recurrence of pterygium after surgical removal. It has also been used topically to prevent corneal vascularization after chemical burns.

Adverse Effects

The drug is radiomimetic and is highly toxic to the hematopoietic system when given systemically. Other possible side effects include vomiting, anorexia, headache, and allergic reactions. There are no significant systemic side effects with topical therapy, changes in skin pigmentation of eyelids have occurred in blacks. Occlusion of the lacrimal puncta may occur.

Dosage

The drug is prepared in 15 mg vials. As prophylaxis against recurrence of pterygium, a 1:2000 solution is applied to the eye every 3 hours during the day for 6 to 8 weeks. Treatment is started within a few days after surgical removal of the pterygium.

INFLIXIMAB

Description

Infliximab is a chimeric anti-TNF-alpha monoclonal antibody containing a murine TNF-alpha binding region and human IgG1 base. It has been approved for the treatment of psoriasis, Crohn's disease, ankylosing spondylitis, psoriatic arthritis, rheumatoid arthritis and ulcerative colitis. It has also been tried successfully in various ocular conditions.

Ophthalmic Uses

It has been effectively used for managing the refractory uveoretinitis in Behçet's disease, noninfectious scleritis, severe ocular rheumatoid disease, scleromalacia perforans, neovascular age-related macular degeneration, Vogt-Koyanagi-Harada disease, retinal vascular tumors, refractory retinal vasculitis due to sarcoidosis, diffuse subretinal fibrosis syndrome, idiopathic sclerosing orbital inflammation (myositis) when given along with methotrexate and for sight threatening thyroid associated ophthalmopathy.

Adverse Effects

Lymphoma and other malignancies, some fatal, have been reported in children and adolescent patients treated with TNF blockers. Reactivation of latent tuberculosis and increased incidence of opportunistic infections has been seen. Infusion related reactions and hepatitis also has been reported in some cases.

Preparation and Dosage

- 100 mg vial of infliximab is available.
- Infliximab is administered by 5 to 10 mg/kg by intravenous infusion at 6–8 week intervals.

IMIQUIMOD
(Aldara)

Description

It is an immunomodulator drug. It is available as 5% cream for local application.

Indications

1. Confirmed cases of superficial basal cell carcinoma (sBCC) less than or equal to diameter of 2 cm if surgery is not feasible.
2. Typical, nonhyperkeratotic, nonhypertrophic actinic keratoses.

Contraindications

It should not be used in patients with immunocompromised status or autoimmune diseases.

Precautions

Sunlight exposure should be avoided as there is high chance of sunburn with imiquimod cream. Enough studies are not there regarding use in pregnancy so should be used with caution.

Dosage and Administration

The cream is applied twice a week for 16 weeks. It should be applied at night so that it remains on the applied skin for eight hours before washing with mild soap and water. Before applying the area should be dry and clean.

Adverse Effects

Reactions at the applied area such as itching, rash, erythema, burning pain are common. Other adverse effects can be flu like symptoms such as upper respiratory tract infections, sinusitis, rhinitis, headache, back pain, fever, lymphadenopathy, chest pain, nausea, myalgia, etc.

VINCRISTINE
(Brand name: Oncovin)

Description

It is a mitotic inhibitor, and is used in cancer chemotherapy.

Action

It binds to tubulin dimers, inhibiting assembly of microtubule structures.

Ophthalmic Uses

Vincristine is used for the treatment of retinoblastoma, primary intraocular lymphoma, orbital lymphomas, neuroblastoma and rhabdomyosarcoma.

Side Effects

The common side effects of this drug include nausea and vomiting, stomach pain and cramps, constipation/diarrhea and thinned or brittle hair.

The main serious side-effects of vincristine are peripheral neuropathy, hyponatremia, constipation and hair loss.

Dosage and Administration

The dose of Vincristine sulfate Injection is 1.4 mg/m² for adults and 1.5–2 mg/m² for pediatric patients. The drug is administered intravenously at weekly intervals. Chemotherapy is usually given as a course of several sessions (cycles) of treatment over a few months. The number of cycles will depend on the type of cancer being treated.

Caution should be exercised in patients with hepatic dysfunction.

ETOPOSIDE (TOPOSAR, VEPESID)

Description

Etoposide is a chemotherapy drug derived from a type of plant alkaloid known as a *podophyllotoxin*.

Action

It blocks cells in the late S-G2 phase of the cell cycle. It is thought to work by blocking the action of an enzyme in cells called topoisomerase II. Cells need this enzyme to keep their DNA in the proper shape when they are dividing into 2 cells. Blocking this enzyme leads to breaks in the DNA, which leads to cell death. Because cancer cells divide more quickly than normal cells, they are more likely than normal cells to be affected by etoposide.

Dosage and Administration

Etoposide can either be given as an injection into a vein or taken by mouth as a capsule. It is administered in a dosage of 100 mg/m^2 intravenously for 5 days in adults. The pediatric dosage for retinoblastoma is 150 mg/m^2 IV 3 weekly for 9 cycles.

Ophthalmic Uses

It is one of the first line drugs for the treatment of retino-blastoma.

Side Effects

Documented hypersensitivity; myelosuppression; liver impairment; IV administration may cause death.

CYCLOSPORINE
(Sandimmune, Restasis ophthalmic emulsion)

Description

It is a cyclic polypeptide that suppresses some humoral immunity and, to a greater extent, cell-mediated immune reactions such as delayed hypersensitivity.

Action

It is a calcineurin inhibitor.

Dosage and Administration

It is given in an oral dosage of 5–7 mg/kg/day in a single or two divided doses. Topical cyclosporine is used in the concentrations of 0.05%, 1% and 2% concentrations. Exact concentration and frequency of administration depends on the disease being treated and its severity.

Ophthalmic Uses

Systemic cyclosporine is used in retinoblastoma, for prevention and treatment of rejection in high risk corneal transplantations.

Topical cyclosporine has been used in dry eye, vernal keratoconjunctivitis and post corneal transplantation.

Side Effects

The principal adverse reactions of systemic cyclosporine therapy are renal dysfunction, tremor, hirsutism, hypertension,and gum hyperplasia. Hypertension, which is usually mild to moderate, may occur in approximately 50% of patients.

Ophthalmic emulsion (Restasis®) mainly causes ocular burning and conjunctival hyperemia.

Anti-VEGF Agents

RANIBIZUMAB
(Lucentis)

Description

Ranibizumab is a recombinant, fully humanized monoclonal anti-VEGF(vascular endothelial growth factor)-A antibody available as 10 mg/ml solution in a single-use vial for intravitreal injection. Its molecular weight is 49 kD.

Indication

It is used in neovascular (wet) form of age-related macular degeneration (AMD).

Mechanism of Action

It prevents the interaction of VEGF,which is an angiogenic factor, with the endothelial cells thus inhibiting cellular proliferation, new vessel formation and vascular leakage.

Adverse Effects

Conjunctival hemorrhage, eye pain, vitreous floaters, increased intraocular pressure, and intraocular inflammation are the common adverse effects.

Precautions

Endophthalmitis, retinal detachment and thromboembolic events may occur. Intraocular pressure should be monitored as there is risk of increased IOP.

Contraindications

It is contraindicated in presence of ocular or periocular infections and hypersensitivity to any of the ingredients in the formulation. Also contraindicated in patients who have a history of having had thrombo embolism/stroke.

Dose and Administration

Ranibizumab 0.5 mg (0.05 mL) is administered by intravitreal injection once a month. Later, if once a month injection is not feasible, it can also be administered once every three months, though this reduces the efficacy.

PEGAPTANIB SODIUM
(Macugen)

Description

Pegaptanib sodium is available as a single-use glass syringe pre-filled with 0.3 mg the drug for intravitreal injection its molecular weight is 50 kilodaltons (kD)

Indication

It is used in neovascular (wet) form of age-related macular degeneration (AMD).

Mechanism of Action

Pegaptanib is an aptamer, a pegylated modified oligonucleotide, which binds selectively with the extracellular vascular endothelial growth factor (VEGF). This leads to inhibition of VEGF which is an angiogenic factor responsible for increased vascular permeability and inflammation in neovascular (wet) form of age-related macular degeneration (AMD).

Adverse Effects

Anterior chamber inflammation, blurred vision, cataract, conjunctival hemorrhage, pain, increased intraocular pressure (IOP), punctate keratitis, reduced visual acuity, vitreous floaters and opacities may occur.

Precautions

Patients should be monitored for increased intraocular pressure and for endophthalmitis associated with intravitreal pegaptanib injection.

Contraindications

It is contraindicated in presence of ocular or periocular infections and hypersensitivity to any of the ingredients in the formulation.

Dose and Administration

Pegaptanib 0.3 mg should be administered once every six weeks by intravitreal injection into the affected eye.

BEVACIZUMAB
(Avastin)

Description

Bevacizumab is a recombinant humanized monoclonal antibody which binds to the human vascular endothelial growth factor (VEGF). It inhibits the binding of VEGF to its receptors, Flt-1 and KDR, on the surface of endothelial cells. Though not approved by FDA for intraocular use, it is used off-label on the basis of clinical studies as intravitreal injection for treatment of a number of vascular and retinal problems. It has recently been shown to have antifibrotic properties. It has a greater molecular weight (149kD) compared to Ranizumab or Pegaptanib.

Adverse Effects

These are mainly due to inherent risks of the intravitreal injections including hemorrhage, pain, reduced visual acuity, floaters, endophthalmitis, etc.

Indications

Has been used successfully in choroidal neovascularisation, proliferative diabetic retinopathy, neovascular glaucoma, diabetic macular edema, retinopathy of prematurity and macular edema secondary to retinal vein occlusions.

Precautions

Contraindicated in patients who have a history of having had thromboembolism/stroke.

Dosage

It is generally given in the dose range of 1.25 to 2.5 mg (0.05 ml) intravitreal or intracameral injection.

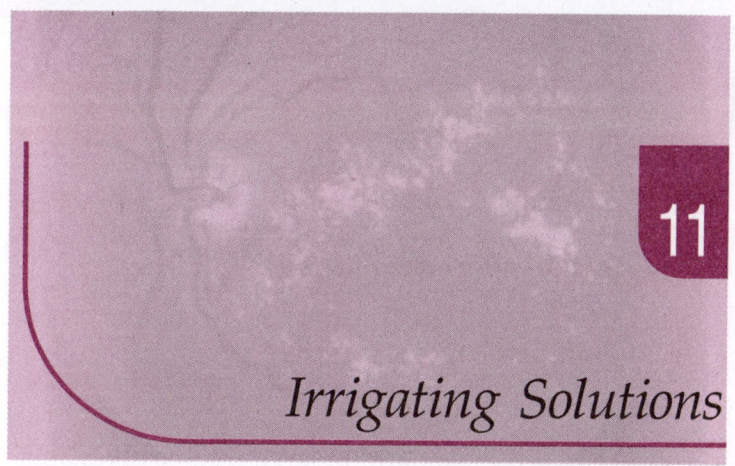

Irrigating Solutions

Irrigating solutions are aqueous solutions and primary purpose of an intraocular irrigating solution is to maintain both the anatomic and physiologic integrity of intraocular tissues. These provide cellular nutrients which are required for intercellular and intracellular function during prolonged intraocular surgery. The major components are sodium, potassium, calcium, magnesium chloride, sodium acetate and citrate. These components help to maintain a thin cornea by avoiding corneal clouding.

An ideal intraocular irrigating solution should:
- Contain concentrations of inorganic and organic constituents similar to those present in aqueous humor and vitreous cavity.
- Not cause corneal edema, corneal endothelium cell loss, crystalline lens opacification, damage to trabecular meshwork and retinal edema.
- Contribute in keeping a normal pressure–volume relationship intraoperatively.

Indications
- Cataract surgery including phacoemulsification and extracapsular cataract extraction.
- Vitrectomy and posterior segment surgeries
- Anterior segment reconstruction.

BALANCED SALT SOLUTION (BSS)
(Intasol)

Composition*

- NaCl 110, KCl 10, $CaCl_2$ 3, Mg Cl_2 1.5, sodium acetate 29, sodium citrate 6
- pH 7.4
- Osmolality 305 mOsm
- BSS 500 ml is the standard for large volume ophthalmic irrigation.

Advantage

Better tolerated irrigant.

Disadvantage

- Lacks the bicarbonate, glucose and glutathione present in aqueous humor.
- Causes a significant decrease in the percentage of corneal endothelial cells (pleomorphism) in longer irrigation.

BALANCED SALT SOLUTION PLUS (BSS PLUS)

Composition*

- NaCl 122.2, KCl 5.8, $MgCl_2$ 0.98, disodium phosphate 3, dextrose 5.11, glutathione(oxidized) 0.30, sodium bicarbonate 25
- pH 7.4
- Osmolality 305 mOsm
- Also known as GBR(glutathione bicarbonate Ringer's) 500 ml enriched with bicarbonate, dextrose and glutathione with basic salts.

Advantage

- It is iso-osmotic with the intraocular tissues.
- Maintains corneal thickness.
- Causes minimal changes in endothelial morphologic characteristics regardless of irrigation time.

- Causes no retinal edema.
- Glutathione helps to protect cells against oxidative stress, maintain integrity of blood aqueous barrier and minimize inflammation.

NORMAL SALINE

Composition*

- NaCl 154
- pH 9.5 7.2
- Osmololality 290 mOsm

Disadvantages

- Not an ideal solution to be used in ophthalmology because causes complete destruction of endothelial cells of cornea within one hour of irrigation.
- Fails to maintain endothelial pump and barrier function resulting in corneal swelling.

PLASMA-LYTE 148

Composition*

- NaCl 86, KCl 5, $MgCl_2$ 1.5, sodium acetate 27, sodium gluconate 23.
- pH 7.4
- Osmolality 299 mOsm

Disadvantages

- It lacks the critical ion, calcium
- Causes the breakdown of junction between the endothelial cells
- Causes corneal edema.

LACTATED RINGER'S SOLUTION

Composition*

- NaCl 102, KCl 4, $CaCl_2$ 3, sodium lactate 28
- pH 6.0 7.2
- Osmolality 277 mOsm

Advantage

Contains most of the essential ions to maintain the integrity of intraocular tissues.

Disadvantages

- Contains 28 mM lactate in a much higher concentration than that present in intraocular fluids.
- Causes various degrees of endothelial cell breakdown and corneal swelling on prolonged perfusion.

S-MA$_2$
Composition*

- NaCl 112.9, KCl 4.8, MgSO$_4$ 1.2, sodium acetate 4.4. sodium citrate 3.4, sodium bicarbonate 25.0, dextrose 8.3
- pH 7.3
- Osmolality 290 mOsm
- It contains glucose, and is buffered by both acetate-citrate and bicarbonate. It is commercially available only in Japan.

Advantages

- It is said to protect corneal endothelium.
- Prevents corneal edema when perfused into the endothelium for extended time period.
- Prevents corneal complication after pars plana vitrectomy.

---

* **(All concentrations are expressed as mMol/litre of the solutions).**

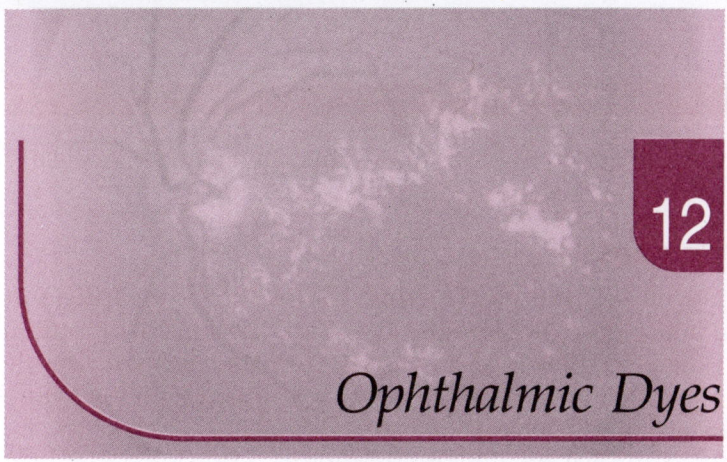

Ophthalmic Dyes

FLUORESCEIN SODIUM STRIPS
(Fluore Stain Strips)

Composition

- Fluoroscein sodium   2%, 4%
- Distilled water qs   100 ml
- Whatman filter paper strip 7 cm × 3 mm

Indications

For staining the anterior segment of the eye when:
- Delineating a corneal injury, herpetic lesion or foreign body.
- Determining the site of an intraocular injury.
- Fitting contact lenses.
- In laser test.
- To ascertain postoperative closure of the corneoscleral wound in delayed anterior chamber reformation.

Directions for Use

Moisten end of strip with a drop of sterile water. Place moistened strip at the fornix in the lower cul-de-sac close to the punctum. For best results, patient should close lid tightly over strip until desired amount of staining is obtained. Another method is to retract upper lid and touch tip of strip to the bulbar conjunctiva on the temporal side until an adequate amount of stain is available for a clearly defined end point reading.

Warnings

Never use fluoroscein while the patient is wearing soft contact lenses because the lenses may become discoloured. Whenever fluorescein is used, flush the eyes with sterile normal saline solution, and wait at least one hour before replacing the lenses.

FLUORESCEIN SODIUM INJECTION

Description

Fluorescein sodium injection is a sterile aqueous solution, available in three strengths 5%, 10% and 25%. Used intravenously as a diagnostic aid. Luminescence in the retina is achieved in 9–15 seconds.

Clinical Pharmacology

The yellowish green fluorescence of the drug demarcates the vascular area under observation distinguishing it from adjacent areas.

Indications and Usage

Indicated in diagnostic fluorescein angiography, indirect ophthalmoscopic assisted angioscopy and iris angiography.

Contraindications

Contraindicated in those persons who have shown hypersensitivity to any component of this preparation.

Precautions

Caution is to be exercised in patients with a history of allergy or bronchial asthma.

Avoid angiography on patients who are pregnant especially those in first trimesters. However, there have been no reports of foetal complications for fluoroscein injection during pregnancy.

Skin will attain a temporary yellowish discoloration, urine attains a bright yellow colour that fades in 24 to 36 hours.

Adverse Reactions

If extravasation occurs it can cause pain in the arm for several hours. Nausea and headache occurs in 10–15% patients after a few minutes of injection of the dye, gastrointestinal distress, syncope, vomiting, hypotension and other symptoms and signs of hypersensitivity have occurred.

Dosage and Administration

Inject contents of the ampoule rapidly into the antecubital vein. In 9 to 14 seconds, luminescence appears in the retinal and choroidal vessels that is observed by standard viewing equipment.

Oral Fluorography

It is done in patients with inaccessible veins where early phase of angiography is not necessary. One gm of fluorescein is given orally and 10–15 minutes are required before the dye is seen in the fundus.

INDOCYANINE GREEN

Description

A water soluble dye with a peak spectral absorption at 8100–810 nm. It contains < 5% sodium iodide.

Composition

- Indocyanine green   25 mg powder
- Distilled water   5 ml

Indication

Used for visualizing choroidal circulation using infrared angiography, because the dye is 98% bound to blood protein, it does not extravasate from the choroidal vasculature.

Directions for Use

It should be dissolved only in distilled water provided because incompatibility with some commercially available water for injection has been reported. Immediately after injection of the dye a bolus of 5 ml of normal saline is injected.

Once dissolved the solution is unstable and must be used within 10 hours.

Warnings

Pregnant and lactating mothers.

Precautions

- In patients allergic to iodides.
- Radioactive iodine uptake studies should not be performed for 1 week after use of Indocyanine Green.

ROSE BENGAL STRIPS

Description

Rose Bengal 1% is a vital stain, which stains dead or degenerated epithelial cells of the cornea and conjunctiva including the nuclei and cell-wall.

Composition

- Rose Bengal   1%.
- Distilled water   95–100 ml.

Indications

For use as a diagnostic agent in routine ocular examination or when superficial corneal or conjunctival tissue change is suspected. Effective aid for the diagnosis of keratitis corrosions or abrasions and for the detection of foreign bodies.

Contraindications

It should not be used in patients with known hypersensitivity to Rose Bengal.

Precautions

To obtain optimal staining and patient comfort, moist the tip of the strip with distilled water, touch the conjunctiva or lower fornix as required with the moistened rose bengal strip. It is recommended that the patient be instructed to blink several times after application as it is highly irritating.

TRYPAN BLUE
(Auroblue, Vision blue)

Description

It is a blue dye (sodium ditolyldisazobis-8-amino-1-naphthol-3, 6-disulfonate) used to stain capsules and has very low toxicity profile. It is available as a 0.1% solution.

Indication

To stain the anterior capsule during capsulorrhexis and in macular hole surgery for maculorrhexis (it stains the internal limiting membrane).

Adverse Effects

It is well tolerated though rare reports of post surgical inflammatory reactions and bullous keratopathy are reported.

Warnings

It is harmful if used systemically as it has been used as an experimental teratogen and may cause liver damage.

Dosage and Administration

It is available as 1 mg single use vials. Each ml contains 0.6 mg trypan blue. It can be injected in the anterior chamber ideally under air bubble and is allowed to stay for a minute to allow staining before removal.

VERTEPORFIN
(VISUDYNE)

Description

It is a photosensitive second generation porphyrin, formulated in a lipid based preparation which augments its solubility in blood. It selectively accumulates in vascular endothelial cells especially the neovascular tissues which have an increased concentration of low density lipoprotein receptors. This dye absorbs light in the infrared range. It is exclusively excreted in stools within 24 hours of administration.

Indication

Verteporfin is indicated for the treatment of classic neovascularisation especially in age-related macular degeneration (photodynamic therapy). The selective uptake and retention of verteporfin in choroidal neovascularisation is important as it limits damage to the surrounding healthy tissues.

Mechanism of Action

After injecting verteporfin, diode laser is used to activate the verteporfin such that the laser causes no thermal damage. The diode laser causes verteporfin to transform from a ground singlet state to an excited triplet state. Thereafter a photochemical reaction ensues, leading to damage of the cells in which verteporfin has accumulated.

Adverse Effects

Ocular: Transient vision disturbance, eye pain, photophobia.

Systemic: Back pain, headache, abdominal pain, dizziness, photosensitivity reaction if exposed to bright light (skin burns). An over dosage will result in prolongation of the period during which the patient remains photosensitive to bright light.

Warnings

While injecting verteporfin avoid extravasation, and if it occurs stop the infusion immediately and apply cold compresses. The site must be protected from direct light until the swelling has faded. Avoidance of bright light > 50 J/cm^2 for at least 5 days after injection. Patient should be encouraged to stay indoors exposed to the ambient indoor light which would help inactivate the drug in the skin through photo bleaching.

Contraindications

Patients with porphyria or those with known hyper-sensitivity to porphyrin.

Dosage and Administration

- It is commercially available in a single use 15 mg vials as a freeze dried powder that requires reconstitution with sterile water and dilution with 5% dextrose solution. Saline should not be used for dissolving because verteporfin precipitates in saline. It should be used within 4 hours of reconstitution.
- Photodynamic therapy is initiated 15 minutes after the start of the 10 minute verteporfin infusion.
- Dosage is 6 mg/m^2 body surface area.
- The vial should be stored at room temperature and must be protected from sunlight.

13

Chelating Agents

ETHYLENEDIAMINETETRA-ACETATE ACID (EDTA)

EDTA is a chelating agent with a high affinity for many metals. A useful chelating agent in the treatment of band keratopathy and lime injury. The disodium salt in 0.3% sodium is useful after removing corneal epithelium in removing calcium from Bowman's membrane.

Lime injury (e.g. painters) is treated with a similar EDTA preparation. Prompt irrigation of the epithelium-denuded cornea with EDTA should be part of the emergency treatment of alkali burns especially if discrete particles of alkali are superficially embedded within the tissues.

DESFERRIOXAMINE

(Desferal)

Superficial corneal iron deposits may be removed by treatment with a 10% solution (in 1% methylcellulose) four times daily for several weeks. Desferioxamine acts by chelating free iron ions or those that may be loosely attached to the acid mucopolysaccharides of the vitreous.

Clinically it is used for non-surgical chemical removal of iron stains, is applicable to the treatment of small corneal rust stains.

BRITISH ANTILEWISITE (BAL)

British antilewisite is an effective antiarsenic agent that is of definite value in civilian practice as well as in treatment of war gas casualties. BAL treatment reduces corneal damage to only slight residual scarring. The longer the interval between lewisite burn and BAL application, the less effective is the therapeutic effect.

PENICILLAMINE
(Artamin)

This chelating agent for copper, mercury, zinc and lead may be used to treat toxicity from these metals. Another possible use for this drug stems from its ability to prevent cross-linking of collagen fibers. Such cross-linkage is the basis for the tensile strength of the collagen.

ALPHA CYSTEINE

A 0.2 molar solution of cysteine will irreversibly inhibit collagenase. It acts by chelating divalent ions and by disrupting disulfide bonds. It can be used in the treatment of alkali burns.

14

Antiseptics Disinfectants

BETADINE (POVIDONE-IODINE 5% W/V)
(Septidine, Betadine)

Description

It is a broad-spectrum antimicrobial agent with well-established clinical efficacy, and is in use worldwide. Povidone-iodine is an iodophore. An iodophere is a lose complex of elemental iodine with a carrier that serves not only to increase the solubility of iodine, but also to provide a sustained release reservoir of the element. In povidone-iodine, povidone (polyvinyl pyrrolidone) acts as carrier for iodine. The germicidal property of the preparation is due to the presence of elemental iodine, which possess marked antimicrobial action.

Mechanism of Action

Betadine releases elemental iodine slowly from the complex of polyvinyl pyrrolidone. This free iodine is lethal to several strains of bacteria, fungi, protozoa, yeasts and viruses. The spectrum of povidone-iodine (betadine) includes several gram-negative and gram-positive bacteria, fungi, viruses, protozoa and other organisms. Povidone-iodine exerts microbial action against susceptible pathogens.

Properties of Betadine

- Betadine has a broad antimicrobial spectrum.
- Betadine exerts a rapid lethal action against susceptible pathogens killing them within 1 to 2 minutes.
- Pathogens do not develop resistance to betadine.
- Betadine does not lose its activity in the presence of pus, blood and tissue fluid.
- Topical application of betadine does not cause systemic toxicity.
- Supra infection does not develop during therapy with betadine because of its broad antimicrobial spectrum.
- Betadine does not cause sensitization and the incidence of hypersensitivity reaction with betadine is extremely low.
- Betadine is non-irritating to the skin.

Indications

- Eyelids, eyelashes, eyebrows, skin of forehead, cheek, etc. are prepared with diluted solution (betadine-10% with equal amount saline)
- Diluted solution is used to irrigate the eye.

CHLOROCRESOL

This is a potent bactericide. It is used at 0.03 to 0.05% when it is predominantly bacteriostatic. Some people may find this concentration painful on instillation. The solution should be protected from light.

CETRIMIDE

This is a cationic quaternary ammonium compound with an activity similar to benzalkonium chloride. It may be used for preserving eyedrops at a concentration of 0.005%. It is also used for cleansing skin and in contact lens work.

CRESOL

An apparently effective solution for chemical sterilization of sharp instruments contains the following constituents:
- Liquor cresolis compound 8 ml

- Oil of lavender   2 ml
- Thymol crystals   2 g
- Ethyl alcohol   88 ml

This solution is not corrosive to metal instruments and does not dull sharp edges. Surgical instruments experimentally contaminated by bacteria are invariably sterilized within 2 minutes of immersion of this solution and usually within 60 seconds. The thymol and oil of lavender are added to disguise the unpleasant odour of cresol.

ULTRAVIOLET LIGHT

This germicidal properties of ultraviolet light are well known and widely used for sterilization. Before the discovery of antibiotics, UV radiation was successfully employed in treatment of corneal ulcers caused by micro-organisms. Resistance of viruses, fungi and many bacteria to antibiotics and the development of new ultraviolet radiation sources suggest re-evaluation of this old method of therapy. Peak germicidal activity occurs at a wavelength of about 2650 Å (most effective wavelength against bacteria). Nucleoprotein absorption of ultraviolet light has a similar peak, which suggests that the germicidal effect is a result of nucleoprotein destruction. Experimental studies with 2537Å uv light indicates that dosage of 1250 microwatt sec/cm^2 can be tolerated by human cornea in a single dosage without causing permanent scarring. The discomfort of radiation keratitis can be minimized by cycloplegics and topical anesthesia is used before treatment.

ETHYLENE OXIDE

The current belief is that no chemical method will effectively sterilize instruments contaminated with spores with the exception of ethylene oxide. The sharp instruments used in eye surgery tend to be dulled by autoclaving, which was the reason for the past extensive use of sterilizing solutions (which inadequately sterilize spores). Ethylene oxide sterilization has been shown to be efficacious for autoclaving and yet not to damage sharp edges, glass or plastic. This gas, in a concentration of 10 g/L of space will sterilize even resistant organisms and spores within a 2 hours period. Mixing it with hydrocarbon gases eliminates the explosive properties of pure ethylene oxide. The gas is toxic and should be handled with reasonable care. The ethylene oxide gas sterilizer is standard equipment in many hospitals. A small portable sterilizer has been developed and is practicable for private ophthalmic use.

15

Viscoelastics and other Surgical Adjuncts

VISCOELASTICS

Viscoelastics are vital component for any type for intraocular surgery. They help maintain an anatomical situation created by surgeon and maintenance of anterior chamber. They protect corneal endothelium during intraocular surgery from mechanical trauma. They are used to coat implants, instruments and corneal epithelial surface during surgery. They are used to mechanically break synechiae and tamponade bleeding vessels.

General Uses

1. Insertion of lenses for investigative purpose (as gonioscopic solution)
2. Cataract surgery
3. Corneal transplant surgery
4. Glaucoma surgery (viscocanulostomy)
5. Reconstructive surgery following injury
6. As vitreous substitute
7. Topical treatment of dry eye.

SODIUM HYALURONATE
(Hyal, Healon)

Description

Sodium hyaluronate 1%, a large polysaccharide molecule. It is highly viscoelastic and has molecular weight of 1.1–

1.8×10^6. Its viscoelasticity is 100,000–300,000 centipoise. It is obtained from dermis of roster coombs.

Advantage

It is non-allergic and clear, and inhibits phagocytic activity, synthesis and release of prostaglandin by macrophages during phagocytosis. It is nonantigenic.

Indications

- Phacoemulsification with IOL implants
- Facilitates capsulorrhexis.
- Corneal transplant surgery, glaucoma surgery.
- Posterior segment surgeries in the eye.

Adverse Reactions

- Transient postoperative increase in intraocular pressure.
- Corneal edema
- Rarely inflammatory reactions.

Precautions

- Do not overfill the anterior chamber.
- Ensure total removal before surgery.
- Monitor IOP in postoperative phase.

Dose

It is available as 1% (healon), 2.3% (healon 5) and 1.4% (healon GV). Available as preloaded syringe with 27 G or 30 G cannula containing sodium hyaluronate 10 mg/ml or 14 mg/ml strength (in 0.25, 0.50, 0.80, 2 ml and 4 ml syringes).

CHODROITON SULFATE

It is a proteoglycan. It is obtained from shark, bovine, porcine cartilage. The molecular size is $5 \times 100 \times 103$ centistokes. It has low viscosity therefore it cannot maintain space. It is much smaller molecule than sodium hyaluronate. In combination with another biological polymer like sodium hyaluronate, it forms a good viscoelastic. Viscoelastics containing chondroitin sulfate have a negative charge and so are better retained in the anterior chamber.

HYDROXYPROPYL METHYLCELLULOSE
(Viscomet, Appavisc)

Description

It is an artificial compound for use in the eye. Its viscosity is 3000–4000 centipoise approximately and an average molecular weight of 86000, an osmolality of 285 mOsm and a pH of 7.2.

Advantage

Cheap, water soluble, inert, transparent, non-pyrogenic and non-toxic to corneal endothelium.

Indications

Same as sodium hyaluronate.

Adverse Reactions

Same as sodium hyaluronate.

SODIUM HYALURONATE AND CHONDROITIN SULFATE
(Viscoat, Discovisc)

It is highly viscous and less elastic; and is pseudoplastic.

Composition

3% Sodium hyaluronate and 4% chondroitin sulfate with 0.45 mg sodium dihydrogen phosphate hydrate, 2.65 mg disodium hydrogen phosphate and 4.5 ml NaCl (0.5 ml pack).

Indication

Cataract extraction with intraocular lens implantation with poor endothelial count.

Advantage

Effective in protecting endothelium.

Disadvantages

- Does not maintain anterior chamber.
- Difficult to aspirate
- Tends to trap small air bubbles.
- Less cohesive.
- Requires refrigeration.

ENZYMES

ALPHA CHYMOTRYPSIN
(*Alphapsin*)

Description

It is a lyophilized form of crystalline alpha chymotrypsin, a proteolytic enzyme obtained from the pancreas of ox. The diluent is a sterile balanced salt solution to be used for reconstituting the crystals. Package includes one vial alpha chymotrypsin 750 units and a 9 ml vial of diluent.

When instilled into the posterior chamber of the eye, its enzymatic action causes dissolution of zonular fibers attached to the lens.

Indications and Usage

For enzymatic zonulysis in intracapsular lens extraction.

Warnings

Do not use the reconstituted solution if cloudy or if it contains a precipitate. Do not autoclave the powder or the reconstituted solution, excessive heat, alcohol and other chemicals used for sterilization inactivate the enzyme. After the operation discard any unused portion, including the diluent. If the zonules are still intact, irrigate with additional alpha chymotrypsin and wait an additional two minutes before flushing with the diluent.

Precautions

Alpha chymotrypsin may produce an acute rise in intra-ocular pressure following surgery. Use of this preparation is not advised in patients under 20 years of age.

Adverse Reactions

Transient increase in intraocular pressure, moderate uveitis, corneal edema and striation has been reported.

UROKINASE
(Ukidan, Abbokinase)

Description

It is a thrombolytic agent used to dissolve blood clots.

Indication

It is useful for removal of blood clot of hyphema which is then removed with ringer lactate. Microcatheter urokinase infusion has been used to treat central retinal artery occlusion (CRAO).

Contraindication

Ocular infections and ocular malignancy.

Dosage

5000 units of urokinase are dissolved in 2 ml of normal saline and injected into the anterior chamber. Dose for CRAO is 100,000–900,000 IU over 10–90 minutes into the ophthalmic artery.

HYALURONIDASE
(Hyalse)

Description

It is an enzyme that acts by depolymerizing hyaluronic acid, a component of the intercellular ground substance which determines the permeability of tissues.

Indication

Used with local anesthetics for regional anesthesia. It is also used to hasten sub-conjunctival hemorrhage or anterior chamber hyphema.

Contraindication

Ocular infections and ocular malignancy are contra-indication to its use.

Adverse Reactions

It is antigenic and may sometimes produce allergic reactions.

Dosage and Administration

It is available as an odorless powder containing 300 units of activity per mg. For local anesthesia one ampoule of 1500 units is reconstituted with 2% lignocaine and 1 ml of this solution is mixed with the 30 ml vial. The fresh prepared solution rapidly loses activity at room temperature and the solution should be used within 12 hours.

ANTIMITOTIC AGENTS

MITOMYCIN

Description

It is isolated from the fungus *Streptomyces caesopitosus*. It is an antimitotic agent that has weak immunosuppressive properties but is a potent inhibitor of fibroblast proliferation. It is 125 times more potent than 5 FluoroUracil.

Indication

It is useful for glaucoma surgery to prevent postoperative fibrosis. It can be used to prevent recurrence of pterygium after surgery. There is dose response relationship between the concentration and duration of exposure of mitomycin.

The length of exposure is more important than the concentration. It has also been used to prevent reclosure of a stenosed punctum after the snip surgery for punctual occlusion.

Precautions

It should not be allowed to enter the eye as it is very toxic to endothelium.

Adverse Reactions

Long-term topical use can cause persistent epithelial defects and scleral necrosis.

Dosage and Administration

For trabeculectomy a dose of 0.2–0.4 mg/ml is used. Generally the application times vary from 1.3 to 5 minutes. It can be used as 0.01 mg/ml drops for preventing pterygium recurrence.

5-FLUOROURACIL

Description

It is fluorinated analogue of pyrimidine.

Indication

It can be used intraoperatively as well as postoperative subconjunctival injections after trabeculectomy to prevent fibrosis. It has been tried for proliferative vitreoretinopathy associated with retinal detachment.

Precautions

5-FU should be avoided in patients with known corneal disease.

Adverse Reactions

Superficial punctuate keratitis, epithelial defects, filamentary keratitis, and infectious corneal ulcers. Most adverse effects are dose related.

Dose and Administration

- Subconjunctival injections are given as 5 mg/0.5 ml. Injections are given twice a day for the first 7 days followed by once daily for next seven days.
- Intraoperative dose is 50 mg/ml placed under the conjunctival or sclera flap during trabeculectomy.
- 5-FU can also be implanted as a collagen sponge containing 100 micrograms of 5-FU during filtering surgery.

DAUNORUBICIN

Description

Daunorubicin is an anthracycline antibiotic that inhibits cellular proliferation. It is less toxic than mitomycin or fluorouracil. However, its antifibroblastic efficacy is less than mitomycin. It is obtained from *Streptomyces coeruleorubidis*.

Indication

It is used as antifibroblastic agent in glaucoma, pterygium surgery and to prevent proliferation in proliferative vitreoretinopathy (PVR) associated with retinal detachment.

Adverse Reactions

Intravitreal reactions can cause retinal toxicity.

Dosage and Administration

Intraoperative dose is 0.2 mg/ml applied beneath the superficial scleral flap in trabeculectomy. Intravitreal 5 microgram of daunorubicin can be injected to prevent PVR after vitrectomy.

OTHERS

SILICONE OIL
(Aurosil, Adatosil 5000)

Description

It is polymethylsiloxane that is injected into the vitreous space for retinal tamponade in select cases of retinal detachment. Like gas it floats in the eye and takes a superior position.There are two viscosities of silicone oil in use: 1000 mPas and 5000 mPas, the latter has higher density.

Indication

Commonly used for complicated retinal detachments, for prolonged retinal tamponade. However, unlike gases used for tamponade patient can still see through the silicone oil.

Precautions

Its presence can mask ERG response which returns to normal after oil removal. In order to avoid pupillary block glaucoma an inferior iridectomy is performed. When axial length is measured in silicone oil filled eyes, hugely erroneous readings are obtained (> 30 mm).

Adverse Reactions

It can cause cataract, band-shaped keratopathy, peripheral corneal vascularisation and glaucoma. Then it has to be eventually removed. Incidence of glaucoma is 12% over 3 years in silicone oil filled eyes. Because of high index of refraction compared to the vitreous it may induce hyperopia.

CYANOACRYLATE GLUE
(Superglue 1409)

Description

It is an adhesive containing repeating monomers of cyanoacrylate and a hydrocarbon side chain that polymerizes, when in contact with fluids, to solid form. The rate of polymerization depends on the surface area exposed and the pH. It is non-biodegradable.

Indication

It is used for sealing small corneal perforations (< 3 mm) and sometimes for conjunctival button holes allowing time for normal wound healing process to repair the defect. In order to be effective, the glue should be in place for 4–8 weeks. The glue later falls off.

Adverse Reactions

Constant contact with glue can cause mechanical irritation and Giant papillary conjunctivitis (GPC), which requires the use of bandage contact lens. Despite reports of antibacterial properties of the adhesive, the irregularity of the surface can encourage bacterial growth.

FIBRIN GLUE
(Reliseal, Tisseel)

Description

It is a biological tissue adhesive kit comprising of components prepared from plasma and acts as local hemostatic. It is used in ocular surgeries to facilitate healing by helping in adhesion of tissues and prevention of bleeding. The commercially available products are produced from pools of plasma, thus they contain high yields of fibrinogen. The glue comprises of mainly two components, fibrinogen and thrombin. Most of the glues also contain human blood factor XIII and aprotinin. Fibrinogen and thrombin come in contact only after administration and the fibrinogen is activated to form fibrin as in the physiological coagulation cascade. Factor XIII further strengthens the clot by helping in cross-linkage of fibrin. Aprotinin prevents the dissolution of the clot by inhibiting fibrinolytic enzymes and provides stability.

Indications and Usage

It is used in place of sutures in various ophthalmic surgeries (Pterygium, cataract surgery, keratoplasty, squint surgery, treatment of leaking blebs). Like cyanoacrylate glue it can be effective in closure of corneal perforations < 3 mm. It is also used as an adjunct during surgery to control bleeding. It forms a smooth seal along the length of application with less postoperative inflammation and discomfort to the patient compared to cyanoacrylate.

Adverse Reactions

Because of being produced from donated blood, there is a risk of transmitted disease. Autologous donated blood source can be an option to counter the risk.

Precautions

Only thin layer should be applied. Reconstituted material should not be kept for more than prescribed period. Allergic reactions in different grades of severity can occur in susceptible individuals.

Dosage and Administration

The components can be administered simultaneously or one after the other. The glue is applied after thoroughly drying the wound surface and gently pressed for three minutes for making a stable adhesive clot.

HEPARIN

Description

It is a naturally occurring glycosaminoglycan. Pharmacologic heparin is obtained from either bovine lung tissue or porcine intestinal mucosa. It is used to inhibit the coagulation cascade and thereby inhibit postoperative fibrin production.

Indication

To prevent after cataract in pediatric cataract surgery and to prevent reproliferation in proliferative vitreoretinopathy.

Adverse Reactions

Increased intraoperative and postoperative hemorrhage may occur.

Dosage and Administration

It is supplied in vials of 1000 U, 5000 U, 10,000 U. It is added to the infusion in a dose of 5 U/ml. Low mol wt heparin fragments (< 7000 da) are considered superior as the hemorrhagic effects are dissociated from the anticoagulant effects.

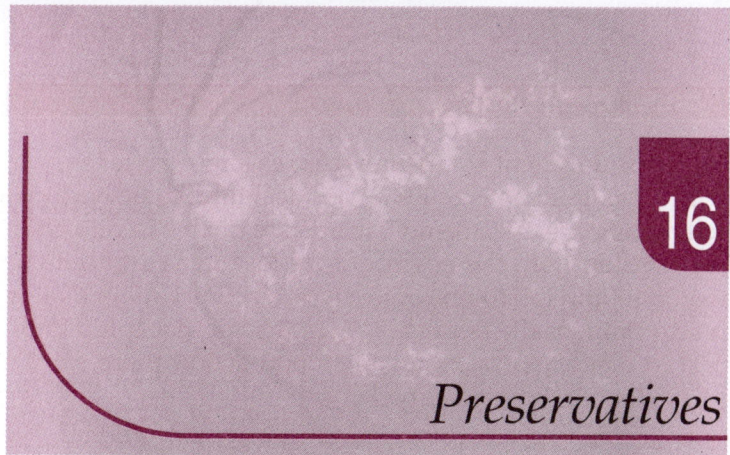

16

Preservatives

In general, preservatives are agents that are added to prevent decomposition. In ophthalmology the term preservative has been used to designate an agent that is added to a preparation or product for the purpose of inhibiting the growth of microorganisms in the preparation, helping to maintain sterility during use.

Two distinct types of preservatives are currently available for commercial use. One group, the surfactants, is ionically charged molecules that disrupt the plasma membrane and are usually bactericidal. The other group of chemical toxins includes mercury and iodine and their derivatives as well as alcohol. These compounds block the normal metabolic process of the cell. Preservative induced ocular toxicity is being increasingly appreciated by ophthalmologists.

BENZALKONIUM CHLORIDE

Benzalkonium chloride is a quaternary ammonium antiseptic with a nitrogenous cationic radical in an ionized molecule.

It has wide specrtum antifungal and antibacterial action. It is an effective inhibitor of bacterial growth of gram positive organisms. The gram negative bacteria are inhibited at conc. 0.005%. Cationic surfactants such as benzalkonium chloride are fairly strong detergents as well as antiseptics. Benzalkonium acts as a bacteriostatic and bacteriocidal agent by virtue of decreasing surface tension, with a resultant change in the permeability of the bacterial cell membrane. As a result bacteria are unable to remain in equilibrium with the environment, lose vital intracellular materials and fail to reproduce and survive. Unfortunately it also changes the permeability of the corneal epithelium, and at conc. necessary for microbial action there can be significant corneal toxicity.

It is used as an antiseptic in many commercial eye preparations in weak concentrations (1:7500 to 1:50,000). It is considered as the preservative of choice. Its efficacy is enhanced in the presence of EDTA thus allowing a lower concentration to be used

Benzalkonium chloride (BAC) stronger than 0.1% may produce skin irritation. It cannot be used in soft contact lens solutions. Soft lens bind large amount of Benzalkonium chloride during soaking and when lens is placed on the eye, BAC is rapidly released, generating a toxic conc. of BAC in the tears. In hard contact lens preparations the 0.01% concentration tends to produce ocular irritation. For this reason, most hard contact lens solutions preserved with this agent contain 0.004% BAC.

CHLORBUTANOL

A less commonly used ophthalmic preservative is chlorbutanol, generally present in ophthalmic preparation at a conc. of 0.155–0.5%. It is fungistatic as well as bacteriostatic against both gram-positive and gram-negative organisms. Chlorbutanol is often formulated together with BAC. The efficacy of these two preservatives is enhanced when they are used together. Chlorbutanol is also often combined with EDTA in ophthalmic drug formulations.

For stability, chlorbutanol must be formulated at a pH below 6 and it can not be autoclaved. It accumulates in soft lenses and is suitable only for hard lens products.it has been found to disrupt the corneal epithelial barrier, leading to epithelial edema and punctuate staining.

METHYL AND ETHYL PARABENS

Esters of parahydroxy benzoic acid (methyl and ethyl parabens) are more effective against molds and fungi than against bacteria. They affect gram-positive more than gram-negative bacteria. Their major drawn backs are that they show only limited effectiveness against *Pseudomonas aeruginosa* and they are less capable with many chemicals including polyxin pyrrolidone and methyl cellulose. They can sometimes produce allergic reactions and are unstable at high pH. Occasionally used in artificial tears and non-medicated ointments in a concentration of 0.02–0.18%.

CHLORHEXIDINE DIGLUCONATE

Chlorhexidine is a diguanide chemically arranged such that it does not intercalate readily into the phospholipid membrane. It is useful as an antimicrobial agent in the same range of concentrations as is benzalkonium chloride. It is more effective against gram-positive organisms and has limited action against fungi. It has high propensity to react with many therapeutic and diagnostic agents and so is routinely used in contact lens care solutions (0.005%) rather than in eyedrops.

EDTA

Disodium ethylenediaminetetraacetic acid (EDTA) is a special type of molecule known as a chelating agent. Its role in preservation is to assist the action of thiomersal, benzalkonium chloride and other agents. By itself, EDTA does not have a highly toxic effect on cells.

THIOMERSAL

Organic mercurial form a group of antimicrobials with both antibacterial and antifungal effects. Thiomersal, phenylmercuric acetate and phenyl mercuric nitrate are among the antimicrobials in this group. They act by releasing mercury, which interferes with respiratory enzymes of the microbes. The mercury released may cause mercurialentis, a graying of the crystalline lens on prolonged use. Mercurialentis is asymptomatic and does not usually interfere with vision. Thiomersal at 0.005% the concentration most frequently used in ophthalmic preparations, has not been found to cause mercurialentis, perhaps due to its greater stability and solubility.

EDTA potentiates the action of thiomersal whereas the action of either phenyl mercuric acetate or nitrate is not. Although soft lenses absorb thiomersal, this preservative does not bind to, and thus build up in soft lenses. It can however bind to proteinaceous debris on the lenses. Thiomersal must be formulated at an alkaline or neutral pH. It has no known effect on tear film stability.

PHENYL MERCURIC NITRATE/ACETATE

This possesses both antibacterial and antifungal activity. Although, its activity against *Pseudomonas aeruginosa* is not very marked, it is the best of three recommended preservatives (viz. Phenyl mercuric nitrate or acetate, 0.002% Benzalkonium chloride 01% or 0.2% chlorhexidine acetate, 0.01%) and is the agent of choice for fluorescein drop. The antibacterial activity is unaffected by changing pH. The solution should be protected from light. There is a possibility that metallic mercury may deposit on standing. It should not be used in drops which are intended for long-term use as there is the danger of mercurialentis. Sensitization may occur to phenyl-mercuric nitrate. As a preservative in eyedrops a conc. up to 0.002% is used.

POLYQUAD

It is used in both soft and RGP lens formulations. Polyquad is similar to BAC in composition and action but has minimal adverse effects. It has a high molecular weight that prevents it from being absorbed into the contact lens matrix.

SODIUM PERBORATE

Sodium perborate was one of the first oxidative-type preservatives to be used. It causes oxidative damage to microbial cell membranes, alters the protein synthesis, and disrupts enzymatic function. On coming in contact with aqueous environment, it releases hydrogen peroxide which is a potent microbicidal making this preservative effective at low concentrations. It has good antibacterial and antifungal activity. While gentler than most other preservatives it may still cause ocular toxicity.

STABILIZED OXYCHLORO COMPLEX (SOC)/PURITE

Stabilized oxychloro complex is a relatively well tolerated, non-irritant preservative. It damages the bacterial protein synthesis by oxidative injury through its oxychloro molecules. It consists of an equilibrium mixture of oxychloro species, predominantly 99.5% Chlorite ($NaClO_2$), 0.5% chlorate ($NaClO_3$) and traces of chlorine dioxide (ClO_2). It has a broad antimicrobial spectrum. It has good safety profile because it disintegrates into components such as sodium chloride, water and oxygen which are normally present in tears. It is being used in various ophthalmic solutions in 0.005% concentration. It is efficacious at low concentrations 0.005%. SOC is safe and well tolerated even when dosed frequently.

SOFZIA™

SofZia is an ionic buffered preservative. It is composed of boric acid, propylene glycol, sorbitol and zinc chloride. Its mechanism of action is similar to oxidizing preservatives. The distinguishing feature is that it actively acts as a preservative in the container but becomes inactive after instillation into the eye when it is exposed to cations that are normally encountered in the tear film of the eye. This is thought to induce fewer corneal changes and less conjunctival inflammation compared with more conventional preservatives such as BAK. It has broad spectrum of antibacterial coverage and is also effective in preventing fungal contamination.

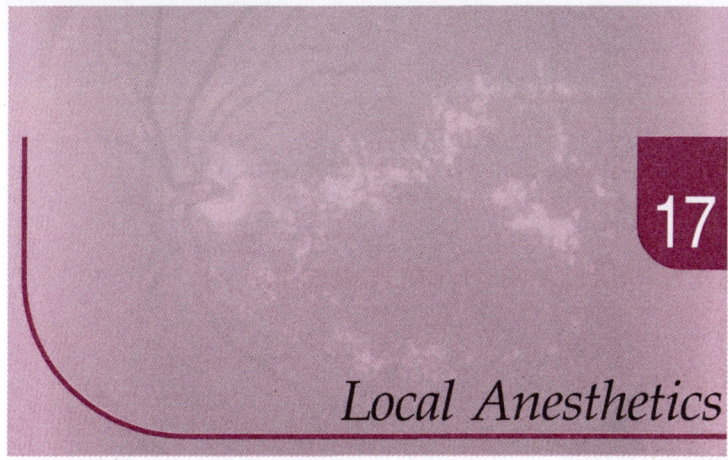

17

Local Anesthetics

PROPARACAINE HYDROCHLORIDE
(Paracaine)

Description

Proparacaine hydrochloride 0.5% is a topical anesthetic prepared as a sterile aqueous ophthalmic solution.

Topical anesthetics stabilize the neuronal membrane and prevent the initiation and transmission of nerve impulses, thereby effecting local anesthesia. The onset of anesthesia usually begins within 20 seconds and lasts up to 15 minutes.

Indications and Usage

For procedures such as in suture removal from the cornea, tonometry, gonioscopy, removal of foreign bodies conjunctival scraping for diagnostic purposes and other short corneal and conjunctival procedures.

Warning

After instillation of this product, the surface of the eye is insensitive and can be scratched without patient feeling it. Eyes should not be rubbed. Do not instill this product repeatedly because severe eye damage may occur.

Dosage and Administration

For tonometry and other procedures of short duration, instill one or two drops just prior to evaluation. For prolonged anesthesia instill one or two drops in the eye (s) every five to ten minutes for three to five doses.

OXYBUPROCAINE HYDROCHLORIDE
(Benoxinate)

Description

Oxybuprocaine, a synthetic derivative from the p-aminobenzoic acid series, possesses a surface anesthetic action, which is 16 times as powerful and a therapeutic ratio, which is 4 times as high as that of cocaine. Oxybuprocaine is distinguished by the following properties:

- It acts rapidly. It thereby reduces waiting time, and permits quicker dispatch of work, especially in diagnostic procedures.
- Oxybuprocaine is gentle on tissues. In this respect oxybuprocaine is unsurpassed by any other similar preparation.
- Oxybuprocaine does not produce cross-sensitization. Patients who are allergic to other para-amino benzoic acid derivatives tolerate oxybuprocaine perfectly well.

Indications and Actions

Oxybuprocaine causes neither hyperemia nor vasoconstriction. It is, therefore, especially suited for diagnostic procedures as well. On the eye, it does not alter pupillary reaction, accommodation or intraocular pressure. If necessary, oxybuprocaine can be combined with epinephrine or with sympathomimetics. It has been found to reduce the miosis during intaocular surgery. This effect is due to its anesthetic action on sensory nerves which inhibit release of a miotic substance.

Dosage and Administration

In ophthalmology, oxybuprocaine is used mainly in the form of the 0.2% solution. Clinical experience, however, revealed that the 0.4% solution while acting more rapidly is just as well tolerated by the tissues. In Tonometry, gonioscopic examination of the irido-corneal angle. Instill 1–2 drops of sterile 0.4% oxybuprocaine and wait for 1 minute. Onset of action occurs after 10–20 seconds and lasts for 15 minutes. Oxybuprocaine solution keeps well when stored in alkali free glassware. They can be sterilized by the usual methods. Owing to the bacteriostatic action of oxybuprocaine the solutions remain aseptic even during use.

LIGNOCAINE HYDROCHLORIDE
(Xylocaine 2%, 4% Drops, 2% Jelly)

Description

A 2% solution of lignocaine is effective at the cornea giving a more rapid, more intense, extensive and prolonged effect. Lignocaine occurs as odourlers crystals, freely soluble as HCl salt in water and is extremely stable.

Mechanism of Action

Lignocaine acts by preventing both the generation and conduction of nerve impulses. The site of action is the membrane. Factors which contribute to the longer duration of anesthetic action are the absence of marked vasodilatation and a resistance of the compound to hydrolysis (this is because of the presence of an amide rather than an ester linkage).

Side Effects

On instillation it causes stinging sensation unlike propracaine. Corneal edema, punctate keratitis, conjunctival hyperemia, lowered tear film break up time, decreased blink reflex, blurred vision, burning sensation and decreased tear secretion (after prolonged use). Less common side effects include decreased wound healing, iritis, blepharitis, conjunctival hemorrhage, corneal ulceration and scarring filamentary keratitis.

Indications

Lidocaine can be used in tonometry, gonioscopy, fundus and contact lens examination, anterior segment examination, contact lens, diagnostic refraction, also for increasing the diagnostic drug effect.

Contraindications

Known hypersensivity to any component of this drug.

Precaution

Lignocaine reacts with certain metals and cause the release of their respective ions, which if injected may cause severe irritation. Adequate precaution should be taken to avoid this type of interaction for instance, prolonged contact between lignocaine solution and metal surfaces (canulas, syringes droppers with metal parts, etc.) may be avoided.

Dosage

For infiltration anesthesia the safe dose is 7 mg/kg body weight with adrenaline and 3 mg/kg body weight without a vasoconstrictor.

Preservative free 1% lidocaine (0.5 ml) ampoules are available for intracameral use during intraocular surgery.

BUPIVICAINE
(Sensoricaine, Marcain)

Description

It is 3–4 times more potent than lidocaine. Bupivicaine is available as 0.75% solution.

Indications

It is used for infiltration anesthesia with 2% lidocaine (50% of 0.75% bupivicaine and 50% of 2% lidocaine along with hyalse).

Precautions

Use lowest dosage that results in effective anesthesia. Avoid intravascular injection. Caution in patients with cardiac arrhythmias, heart block and those in hypotension/shock.

Adverse effects of Infiltration Anesthesia

CNS toxicity: Is dose related. There is restlessness anxiety incoherent speech, lightedness, numbness and tingling of mouth and lips, tremors drowsiness.

CVS toxicity: Myocardial depression, hypotension.

Management of over dosage: Positive pressure by mask. Intravenous diazepam if circulatory depression is present. Intravenous fluids and a vasopressor needs to be administered.

Dosage

The maximum safe dose is 2 mg/kg body weight. Onset of action starts within 5–10 minutes and lasts for 3–5 hours with epinephrine.

ARTICAINE
(Septocaine)

Description

Articaine HCl is an amino amide local anesthetic. It is available as 2% and 4% injection.

Adverse Reactions

Paresthesia, inflammation, headache and pain are commonly reported. Cardiovascular side effects and CNS side effects as restlessness, anxiety, tinnitus, dizziness, blurred vision, tremors, depression, or drowsiness may be due to systemic toxicity.

Precaution

Accidental intravascular injection, methemoglobinemia and hypersensitivity reactions.

Pharmacology

Like other amide local anesthetics it acts by increasing the threshold of nerve excitation and delaying the nerve propagation and rate of rise of action potential. It produces rapid onset of akinesia; is absorbed faster and penetrates tissues effectively. Its fast metabolism makes it less likely to cause systemic side effects.

Indications and Usage

It can be used for ocular surgeries for various types of local, infiltrative or conductive anesthesia including peribulbar, sub-tenon, etc.

18

Other Drugs, Media and Solutions

ADDITIONAL DRUGS

BOTULINUM TOXIN
(Botox)

Description

It is a purified *Clostridium botulinum* neurotoxin of type A. Each vial of Botox contains 100 units neurotoxin complex. It blocks the neuromuscular transmission by inhibiting the release of acetylcholine and reduces the muscle activity.

Indications

It is indicated for the treatment of strabismus and blepharospasm. It is mainly used in those cases which are associated with dystonia, including benign essential blepharospasm or VII nerve disorders. It has been tried in squint for deviations over 50 prism diopters, in restrictive strabismus, in Duane's syndrome with lateral rectus weakness, and also in secondary strabismus caused by prior surgical over-recession of the antagonist. In these cases its efficacy is not well established. It can be used in conjunction with surgical repair to reduce antagonist contracture in chronic paralytic strabismus.

Adverse Effects

Ptosis, superficial punctate keratitis, dry eye, irritation, tearing, lagophthalmos, photophobia, ectropion, keratitis, diplopia and entropion, and local swelling of the eyelid skin can be seen. Other adverse effects are reduced blinking, acute angle closure glaucoma, focal facial paralysis, syncope and exacerbation of myasthenia gravis. Allergic reactions, especially involving skin, can occur. Rarely, serious systemic adverse reactions such as anaphylaxis, arrhythmia, pneumonia, etc. have also been reported. Neutralizing antibody can also develop in rare cases.

Precaution

Should be used with caution in pre-existing neuromuscular disorders. Co-administration of aminogylcosides and curare like drugs with botulinum toxin can increase the risk of neuromuscular weakness. Should not be used in children below 12 years of age.

Contraindications

When there is any infection at the site of injection or when there is hypersensitivity to any of the constituent of the injection.

Dosage

The initial dose is 1.25–2.5 units per site. Can be repeated after three months. The dose can be increased to double in subsequent sessions if the response is not proper in the previous attempt.

TISSUE PLASMINOGEN ACTIVATOR (TPA)
(Activase)

Description

Tissue plasminogen activator (tPA) is a serine protease protein which is involved in breakdown of blood clots. It acts by converting plasminogen into plasmin. It is found generally in the endothelial cells. In the eye it is present in the conjunctiva, cornea, trabecular meshwork, aqueous humor, lens, vitreous and retina.

Indications

The tPA has been used for dissolving the fibrin clots in anterior chamber, in the vitreous after vitrectomy, CRVO, macular hemorrhage and for failed blebs after glaucoma surgery. It has been used after pediatric cataract surgery to prevent fibrinous exudation (more common complication in pediatric group).

Adverse Reactions

At high doses there can be corneal and retinal toxicity apart from hemorrhage and rebleeding. There can be allergic reactions in people sensitive to any of the components in the injection.

Dosage and Administration

Though the half-life of the tPA is about five minutes, it can stay for several hours after intracameral injections in the closed space such as anterior chamber which normally has low daily turnover of the aqueous humor. Doses of 3 µg to 25 µg have been tried in different studies for intracameral injections and an average dose of 10 µg has been seen to produce the desired effects with lesser risk of side effects. Intravitreal injections have also been tried in dose range of 50–100 µg in 0.1 ml. Topical application for clot dissolution in the anterior chamber have shown inconclusive results because of relatively poor penetration of tPA due to large molecular size (68 kDa).

ARTIFICIAL TEARS

COMPOSITION

Polyvinyl alcohol	11.4%
Polyvinyl pyrrolidone	0.6%
Carboxymethylcellulose trehalose	100–200 Mm

Description

They are sterile, soothing, hypotonic solutions for use as a lubricant and as artificial tears.

Actions and Uses

Used to counteract dryness in the absence of natural tears. Also for use as an ocular lubricant to relieve irritation or dryness of the eye due to wind, dry air, smoke, air pollution, etc. Useful as eye drops throughout the day to provide greater comfort and longer wearing of hard contact lenses.

Warnings

If the solution causes eye pain, changes in vision, continued redness or irritation of the eye or if the irritation worsens or relief is not provided within 72 hours, discontinue use and consult a physician.

Directions for Use

Use one or two drops as frequently as required to relieve eye irritation symptoms or as directed by physician.

CORNEAL STORAGE MEDIUM

MODIFIED MCCAREY-KAUFMAN MEDIUM

Description

McCarey-Kaufman modified corneal storage medium is a clear, sterile dextran modified and HEPES buffered tissue culture medium at pH 7.25±0.25 with phenol red indicator, and gentamicin sulfate to protect against bacterial contamination. This medium is capable of storing and transporting human corneas for up to four days at room temperature.

Compostion

It contains Dextran 40, MK powder, HEPES buffer, sodium bicarbonate, phenol red and gentamycin.

Precautions

- Since bacterial contaminations of transplanted cornea have been reported, extreme care should be taken by the user to provide rigidly sterile technique throughout the keratoplasty procedure.
- Each vial should be visually inspected prior to use. The medium should be rose colour in appearance. The change in color to yellow is indicative of possible bacterial contamination and the change in color to red is indicative of a pH change. In any case, any change to either of the above colors should be cause for not using the medium, and it should be discarded, unless the vial is unopened with the original seal intact, in which case it should be returned for evaluation of the problem and replacement.

Storage

McCarey-Kaufman modified storage medium should be stored at 4°–8°C until ready for use.

EYE STORAGE MEDIUM–II

Description

Eye storage medium-II (EP-II) is a product developed with the idea that interrupting the pumping function (bicarbonate pump) of the cornea endothelium prolongs the survival time of the cornea. EP-II can be used for the preservation of not only the whole eye but also the sclerocorneal grafts, being capable of prolonging the survival time of the cornea.

EP-II is a sterile, orange-red clear, slightly viscous aqueous solution adjusted to pH about 7.4 and osmotic pressure about 320 mosm. Amounts of antibiotics added: Crystalline penicillin G potassium-20, 000 units/100 ml and Streptomycin sulfate–0.1 gm (Potency)/100 ml.

Indications

- EP-II interrupts the pumping function (bicarbonate pump) of the corneal endothelium therapy prolonging the survival time of the cornea and maintaining corneal viability for a long time.

- In storing sclerocorneal sections, EP-II is a superior to glucose bicarbonate Ringer solution preservation of the corneal endothelium.
- It has been shown that dextran 70 inhibits swelling of the corneal stroma and protects the corneal endothelium.
- EP-II can be used for preserving not only the entire eye but also the sclerocorneal sections, making possible the prolongation of corneal survival time.

Composition

Each 100 ml of EP-II contains

- Dextran 70   3.5 g
- D. glucose   78.2 g
- Sodium chloride, Potassium chloride, Calcium chloride, Magnesium chloride, Phosphate buffer and Phenol red.......q.s.

OPTISOL

Optisol is a chondroitin sulfate based storage medium. It contains chondroitin sulfate, dextran, optisol base powder, sodium bicarbonate, gentamycin, amino acids, sodium pyruvate, glutamine, mercaptoethanol, ascorbic acid, vitamin B_{12}, adenosine, inosine and purified water. Optisol GS contains streptomycin in addition to these constituents.

Optisol-GS is a 4-degree corneal preservation media which allows up to 14 days preservation. It has been claimed to result in: less stromal edema, fewer Descemet's folds, enhanced endothelial cell preservation, reduced epithelial cell edema, reduced corneal autolysis during storage, minimal rebound swelling. Presence of two antibiotics reduces the risk of endophthalmitis. Corneas stored in Optisol-GS even through 21 days at 4 degrees C have been seen to maintain a high percentage of viable corneal endothelial cells.

DEXSOL

Dexsol also is a chondroitin sulfate based preservation media. *Dexsol contains:* Chondroitin sulfate, dextran 40, dexsol base powder, sodium bicarbonate, gentamycin, amino acids, sodium pyruvate, L-glutamine, mercapto-ethanol and purified water.

Corneas have been shown to have significantly fewer morphologic changes after 14 days at 4°C in the Optisol-medium than in the DexSol-medium. The Optisol-stored corneas were also seen to be significantly thinner than those stored in DexSol for a 5-hour period at 37°C after 14 days of storage at 4°C.

CONTACT LENS SOLUTIONS

HARD CONTACT LENS SOLUTIONS

Ingredients	Preservative	Category	Directions for Use
Polyoxyl 40 stearate times Polyethylene glycol 300	Chlorobutanol	Cleaning and rewetting solution	1–2 drops up to 6 times a day
Phenyl mercuric nitrate (0.004%)		Cleaning solution	Fill storage case with enough and solution leave for 4 hours
Polyvinyl alcohol	Thiomersal, EDTA 0.01%	Lubricating and rewetting solution	—
Polyvinyl alcohol HPMC.	Edetate disodium, Benzalkonium chloride (0.004%) with water	Wetting solution	Apply to both surface of the lens and rub between thumb and forefinger and rinse
Purified water	Edetate disodium (0.25%) Benzalkonium chloride	Soaking solution and leave	Fill the storage case for 4 hours
—	Chloride 0.01% Edetate disodium 0.2%	Cleaning and soaking solution	—

Contd...

Contd...

Ingredients	Preservative	Category	Directions for Use
Non-ionic surfactant	0.004% THIM	Cleaning solution	–
Distilled water, sodium chloride, Pot. chloride, HEC, Boric acid, Poloxamer 407	Edetate disodium 0.05%	Lubricating rewetting solution	1 or 2 drops to be put on lens 5–6 times
Purified water NaCl, Polyethylene glycal, KCL HEC Poloxamer 407	Edetate disodium 0.05% Benzalkonium chloride 0.01%	Purpose	Wet with one drop on each side of lens

SOFT CONTACT LENS SOLUTIONS

Ingredients	Preservative	Category	Directions for Use
1. Twin 21, Polymeric cleaning agent.	THM and Edetate disodium.	Daily cleaning solution	Put the lens in your palm, put two drops and rub for 20 seconds.
2. Sodium chloride, Boric acid, Sodium Borate.	–	Preserved saline solution	–

Contd...

Contd...

Ingredients	Preservative	Category	Directions for Use
3. Sodium chloride 0.9%	–	Rinsing solution	–
4. Sodium chloride, Sod. Phosphate.	Edetate disodium 0.1% Thiomersal 0.001%	Rinsing and storage solution	–
5. Sod. Chloride, Povidone Octyl Phenaxyethanols.	Thiomersal 0.001% EDTA 0.1% Chlorhexidine gluconate 0.005%	Sterile Lubricating solution	–
6. Octyl Phenoxy ethanol HEC, Sod. Chloride Pot. Sorbate 0.13%	EDTA 00 0.35%.	Daily cleaning solution	–
7. NaCl, KCl, Sod. Borate,- HEC Boric acid, Sorbic acid Polyoxamer 407	EDTA solution.	Lubricating and rewetting	–

Index